MEDICAL FINALS

Passing the Clinical

Christopher E. G. Moore BSc MB BS MRCP(UK)
MRC Training Fellow
and Honorary Senior Registrar

Anna M. T. Richardson BSc MB ChB MRCP(UK)
Clinical Registrar

Department of Neurology
Manchester Royal Infirmary
Manchester

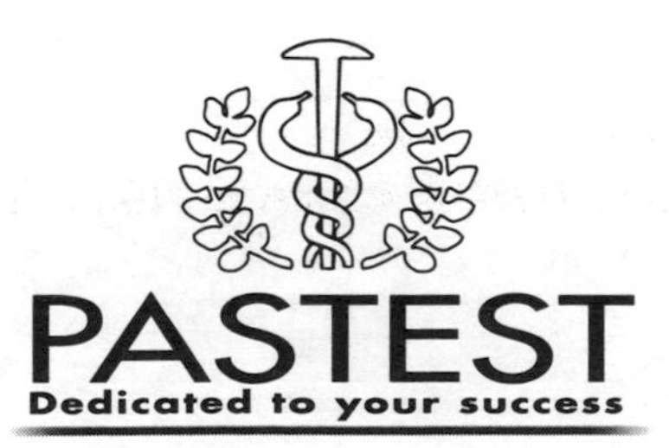

Knutsford
Cheshire
Tel: 01565 752000

First published 1996.

Reprinted 1997, 1998, 1999, 2000, 2001

ISBN 0 906896 43 6

A catalogue record for this book is available from the British Library.

Typeset by Carnegie Publishing, 18 Maynard Street, Preston.
Printed and bound in Great Britain by Biddles Ltd, *www.biddles.co.uk*

CONTENTS

MORE BOOKS FOR MEDICAL STUDENTS FROM PASTEST

FOREWORD

The undergraduate medical curriculum is undergoing dramatic change. However, the ultimate criterion for receiving one's final degree remains a clinical assessment of competence which embraces the ability to obtain a good clinical history and also to elicit physical signs during the examination of patients. Long may this remain the situation and while it does, there is no substitute for exposing undergraduates to as much clinical material as possible because practical experience must be regarded as the cornerstone of good practice.

Nevertheless there is always a learning curve: the pitfalls of interviewing and examining patients are numerous especially when one is inexperienced. This book cannot be regarded as an adequate substitute for seeing as many patients as possible, but it provides valuable supporting information on what to look for when concentrating on single systems or indeed integrating and interpreting signs and symptoms in an holistic way. The text is detailed, comprehensive and aims to guide the student in the clinical exam context. It is instructive and informative and used in conjunction with the regular examination of patients, should lead to success at finals.

A M Heagerty MD FRCP
Professor of Medicine, Manchester Royal Infirmary

ACKNOWLEDGEMENTS

We would like to thank the many colleagues who have given us useful tips whilst producing this book and especially those who have taught us over the years, in particular:

Stephen Brecker, Senior Registrar, Cardiology; Terry Wardle, Consultant Physician; Jon Shaffer, Senior Lecturer, Gastroenterology; George Lipscombe, Senior Registrar, Medicine; Andy Higham, MRC Training Fellow; Matthew Lewis, Registrar, Gastroenterology; Wolfgang Schady, Senior Lecturer, Neurology; Tony Heagerty, Professor of Medicine; Claire Pulford, Lecturer, Geriatric Medicine; Chris Rickards, Senior Registrar, Neurology; David Neary, Professor of Neurology; Eve Russell, Senior Registrar, Psychiatry; Peter Goulding, Consultant Neurologist; Mike Davies, Senior Lecturer in Medicine; Malcolm Littley, Consultant Physician; Mohammed Akil, Senior Registrar, Rheumatology.

Responsibility for the accuracy of the text is of course our own.

We would also like to acknowledge the support of our families; Teddy, Dan, Lucie, Matthew and Keith.

INTRODUCTION

This book is intended for clinical medical students generally and especially for those preparing for their final clinical examination in General Medicine. It is neither a medical textbook nor a clinical methods book. Rather it is an exam-orientated book designed specifically to ensure success in the **Final Clinical MB** examination. It should also prove useful to candidates taking the **PLAB** examination and serve as a primer for the **MRCP** exam.

The clinical exam for the final MB is taken at any time from the beginning of the second clinical year to the last month of the final year depending on the University. Whether psychiatry or paediatrics is included in the exam is also variable. (A guide to the medical approach to a psychiatric long case and four of the most common examples are included in the Long Case section.)

Although some centres do not routinely have a viva-voce examination, all have long and short case exams. The first part of the book concentrates on the **Long Cases**, with a general approach to the Long Case followed by twenty of the more common cases which appear. The second section concentrates on the most popular **Short Cases**; emphasis is given to a structured approach to each type of case. Notes on the format of the **Viva** and how to prepare for it are given in the final section.

It is hoped that the '**Syllabus Checker**' may help pinpoint any areas needing extra work. Although not a definitive list, the most common topics are included and you are encouraged to tick off the cases as you see them and later revise them. Throughout this book cross referencing of case numbers (not page numbers) is indicated by a bold number in brackets, e.g. (**64**) refers you to the case concerning nystagmus.

Remember that, although not its aim, the exam tests your ability to pass exams and not your general doctoring ability. It is therefore important to practise your exam technique alongside learning to be a good doctor.

No pass = No job + No pay + Resit !

As in all first editions there is no doubt room for improvement and we would be grateful for any comments.

ABBREVIATIONS

Most abbreviations used in this book are explained when they first appear. Other common abbreviations are listed below.

ACTH	Adrenocorticotrophin
ALT	Alanine transaminase
AMA	Antimitochondrial antibody
ANA	Antinuclear antibody
AST	Aspartate transaminase
CABG	Coronary artery bypass graft
CVA	Cerebrovascular accident
dsDNA	Double stranded DNA
FBC	Full blood count
FSH	Follicular stimulating hormone
HbA_1	Haemoglobin A_1
HbA_{1C}	Glycosylated haemoglobin
HOCM	Hypertrophic obstructive cardiomyopathy
LFTS	Liver function tests
LH	Luteinising hormone
MCS	Microscopy, culture, sensitivity
MCV	Mean cell volume
RA	Rheumatoid arthritis
RhF	Rheumatoid factor
SIADH	Syndrome of inappropriate ADH
SLE	Systemic lupus erythematosus
SMA	Smooth muscle antibody
TIA	Transient ischaemic attack
TFT	Thyroid function test

NORMAL VALUES

Albumin	35–55 g/l
Alkaline phosphatase	30–130 iu/l
Aspartase amino-transferase	5–27 iu/l
Bicarbonate	24–30 mmol/l
Bilirubin	2–13 μmol/l
Calcium	2.15–2.65 mmol/l
Chloride	93–108 mmol/l
Creatinine kinase	0–170 iu/l
Creatinine	55–125 μmol/l
Erythrocyte sedimentation rate	0–10 mm (1st hour)
Gamma GT	0–30 iu/l
Haemoglobin (males)	13.5–17.5 g/dl
Haemoglobin (females)	11.5–15.5 g/dl
Mean corpuscular volume	76–98 fl
Phosphate	0.80–1.4 mmol/l
Platelet count	150–400 × 10^9/l
Potassium	3.8–5 mmol/l
Sodium	136–149 mmol/l
Thyroid-stimulating hormone	0.8–3.6 mU/l
Thyroxine	70–160 nmol/l
Total protein	65–80 g/l
Urea	2.5–6.5 mmol/l
Vitamin B_{12}	200–900 pg/ml
White blood count	4–11 × 10^9/1

SYLLABUS CHECKER

As an aid to revision you can use this syllabus as your own personal checklist. You should aim to achieve at least two ticks per case before the date of the examination.

			Read	Seen/Taught on	Happy with
LONG CASES					
	1	Myocardial infarction			
	2	Infective endocarditis			
	3	Bronchial carcinoma			
	4	Chronic bronchitis / Emphysema			
	5	Cystic fibrosis			
	6	Chronic liver disease			
	7	Inflammatory bowel disease			
	8	Rheumatoid arthritis			
	9	Systemic lupus erythematosus			
	10	Chronic renal failure			
	11	Nephrotic syndrome			
	12	Multiple myeloma			
	13	Diabetes			
	14	Hyperthyroidism / Graves' disease			
	15	Depression			
	16	Psychosis / schizophrenia			
	17	Anorexia nervosa			
	18	Substance abuse			
	19	Stroke			
	20	Multiple sclerosis			
SHORT CASES					
CVS	21	Mitral stenosis			
	22	Mitral regurgitation			
	23	Aortic stenosis			
	24	Aortic regurgitation			

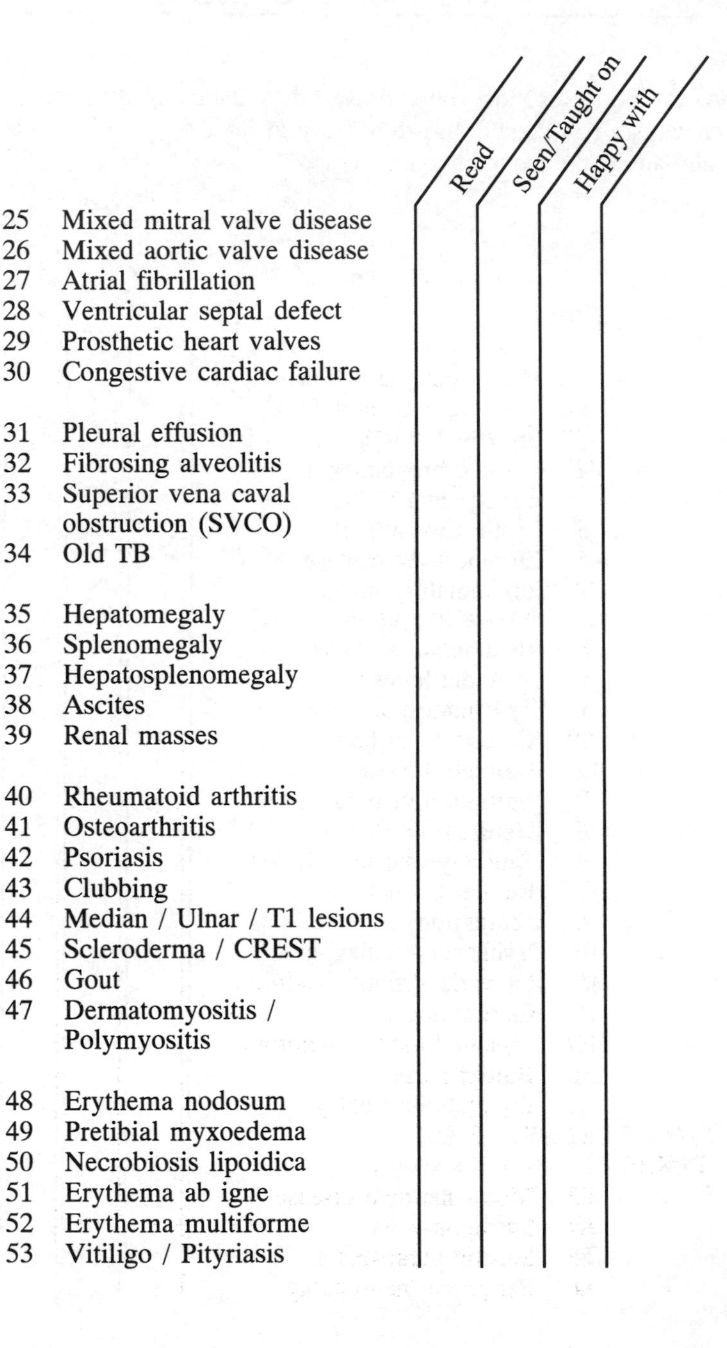

25 Mixed mitral valve disease
26 Mixed aortic valve disease
27 Atrial fibrillation
28 Ventricular septal defect
29 Prosthetic heart valves
30 Congestive cardiac failure

RS

31 Pleural effusion
32 Fibrosing alveolitis
33 Superior vena caval obstruction (SVCO)
34 Old TB

ABDO

35 Hepatomegaly
36 Splenomegaly
37 Hepatosplenomegaly
38 Ascites
39 Renal masses

HANDS

40 Rheumatoid arthritis
41 Osteoarthritis
42 Psoriasis
43 Clubbing
44 Median / Ulnar / T1 lesions
45 Scleroderma / CREST
46 Gout
47 Dermatomyositis / Polymyositis

SKIN

48 Erythema nodosum
49 Pretibial myxoedema
50 Necrobiosis lipoidica
51 Erythema ab igne
52 Erythema multiforme
53 Vitiligo / Pityriasis

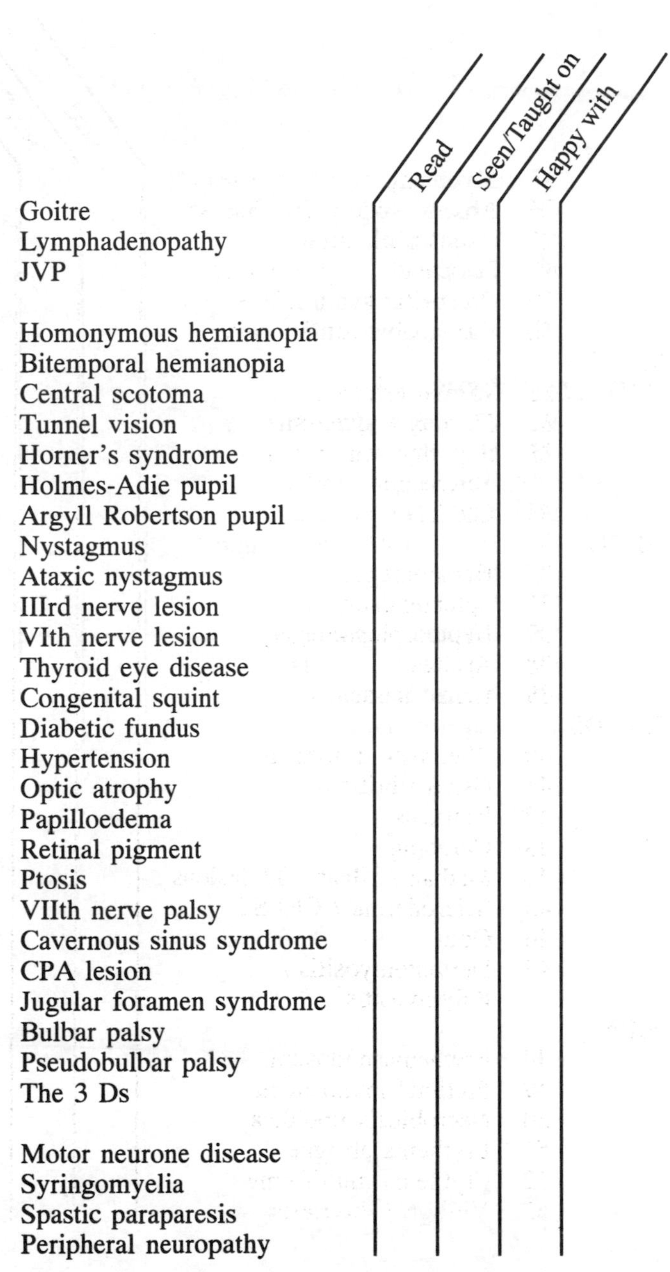

NECK

54 Goitre
55 Lymphadenopathy
56 JVP

CNS

57 Homonymous hemianopia
58 Bitemporal hemianopia
59 Central scotoma
60 Tunnel vision
61 Horner's syndrome
62 Holmes-Adie pupil
63 Argyll Robertson pupil
64 Nystagmus
65 Ataxic nystagmus
66 IIIrd nerve lesion
67 VIth nerve lesion
68 Thyroid eye disease
69 Congenital squint
70 Diabetic fundus
71 Hypertension
72 Optic atrophy
73 Papilloedema
74 Retinal pigment
75 Ptosis
76 VIIth nerve palsy
77 Cavernous sinus syndrome
78 CPA lesion
79 Jugular foramen syndrome
80 Bulbar palsy
81 Pseudobulbar palsy
82 The 3 Ds

LIMBS

83 Motor neurone disease
84 Syringomyelia
85 Spastic paraparesis
86 Peripheral neuropathy

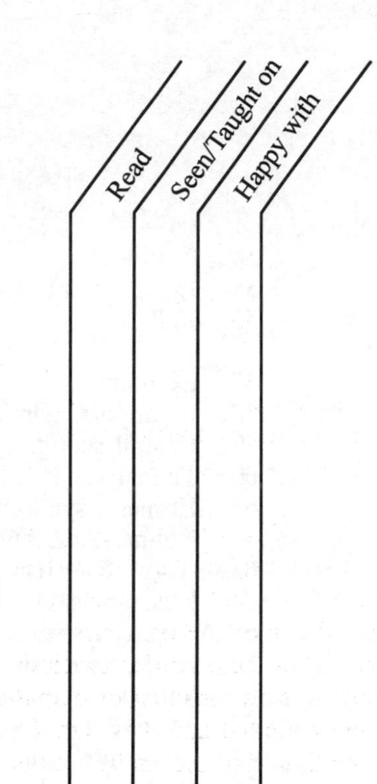

87 Myopathy
88 Absent ankle jerks and extensor plantars
89 Pes cavus
90 Cerebellar syndrome
91 Gait abnormalities

SPOT DIAGNOSES

92 Cushing's syndrome
93 Hypothyroidism
94 Acromegaly
95 Addison's disease
96 Hereditary haemorrhagic telangiectasia
97 Parkinson's disease
98 Myotonic dystrophy
99 Myasthenia gravis
100 Neurofibromatosis
101 Paget's disease

INTRODUCTION TO THE LONG CASE

Candidates are usually given 45–60 minutes to take a history from and examine a patient, followed by 15 minutes for presentation and discussion. Do not be surprised if you are taken back to the patient to demonstrate the physical signs you have elicited.

Do ensure that you allow yourself at least 5 minutes at the end to prepare yourself and your notes before being taken in to see the examiners. Write a summary of the salient features in the history and on examination and your differential diagnosis. It is wise to prepare in advance a list of the investigations you would perform together with appropriate treatment as these are the questions most likely to be asked by the examiners.

It is important to establish a good rapport with the patient. Introduce yourself, explain how important the examination is to you, what you have to do and how much time you have. Try to make the patient feel that they are on your side against the examiner, this way they will try to help you as much as possible early on. Find out if the patient is an inpatient or outpatient. If an inpatient find out when they were admitted and why. Often patients in the exam have chronic conditions and are under routine follow-up: in these cases the presenting complaint may go back many years and it is best to go over the history chronologically and then concentrate on the major current problems.

Don't forget to ask the patient if they know their diagnosis!

Remember, you are expected to perform a full physical examination, including measurement of blood pressure and urinalysis. Occasionally the patient in the long case will have no abnormal physical signs.

The examiners might expect you to present the case fully – be clear and concise, avoiding long lists of negative findings. Volunteer a short summary at the end rather than waiting to be asked. Be prepared however for the examiner instead to plough straight in with questions regarding your differential diagnosis and management plan.

A good start may be one such as this, *"I have been to see Mrs Smith, a 53 year old lady, who is currently an inpatient at this hospital under the care of Professor Jones"*. Then either, *"She was well until two weeks ago when she presented with acute central chest pain . . ."* or *"She has a 15 year history of rheumatoid arthritis and was admitted last week for investigation of anaemia . . ."*.

Be courteous at all times – to patients and examiners alike!

LONG CASE INDEX

Listed below are popular long cases which appear frequently in exams. Those in **bold** are included in the long case section in this book as they are the most common / important.

THE LONG CASE

Presenting Complaint (PC)
History of the Presenting Complaint (HPC)
Past Medical History (PMH)
Family History (FH)
Drug History (DH)
Review of Systems (ROS)
Social History (SH)
Clinical Examination
Summary

PC Remember to use the patient's words – not your interpretation of them. Patients rarely complain of melaena / haemoptysis / dysarthria etc!

HPC For each symptom complained of you need to ascertain the following:
Onset – sudden or gradual
Duration
Pattern – continuous or episodic. If episodic the frequency and duration of individual episodes.
Course of illness to date – Static / Progressive / Improving
Precipitating / Aggravating / Relieving factors
Associated symptoms

Once you have questioned the patient fully regarding PC, specifically ask the other questions relating to that particular organ system.
E.g. If patient complains of shortness of breath and cough, ask specifically about Sputum / Haemoptysis / Fever / Chest pain.

PMH Straightforward
Ask specifically about past Medical / Surgical / Psychiatric histories.
Ask specifically about Hypertension / Diabetes / Asthma / TB / Rheumatic fever.

FH Record details of all first degree relatives (Parents / Siblings / Children)
Record: Age at death / Cause of death / Related illnesses

DH Use proprietary names rather than brand names.
Record: Dose / Dose frequency / Duration of prescription
Recent changes in medication especially those made during this inpatient stay?

Ask specifically about allergies and their nature.

ROS Briefly ask questions pertaining to each organ system.
Always ask about Weight loss / Appetite / Fever / Rash / General wellbeing.

SH Smoking habit
Smoker / Ex-Smoker / Life-long Non-Smoker

Alcohol consumption See (**18**) for more details
Occupation and previous occupations / Unemployment
Marital status Married / Single / Divorced / Widowed
Dependants
Wage / Income support / Invalidity benefit / Other allowances
House / Bungalow / Flat / Steps
Driving ability
Activities of daily living Washing
Dressing
Eating / Eliminating
Shopping
Socialising

Home Help / District Nurse

EXAMINATION

For the long case you will be expected to perform a **full** physical examination, including **Blood pressure** and **Urinalysis.** Although examination techniques for all the relevant systems are included in this book, you need to devise your own routine and be comfortable with it, avoiding unnecessary repetition and ensuring nothing is missed out.

For example:

General Appearance	Well / Unwell / Febrile Distressed / Dyspnoeic / In pain Pale / Jaundiced Cachectic / Obese

Hands
Face
Neck
Chest (CVS/Resp)
Abdomen
Nervous system
Musculoskeletal system

Urinalysis

CASE 1: MYOCARDIAL INFARCTION

Appears fairly frequently as a long case; it is a common condition and patients are usually relatively well and able to give a clear story.

PC **Chest pain** (usually)
Sometimes no chest pain but shortness of breath (SOB)
Collapse / Sweating

HPC Pain **Central** / Radiation to Neck / Jaw / Teeth / **Arms** (one or both, usually LEFT)
Crushing / Squeezing / Tight / 'Like a band'
Occasionally felt as radiation only (no pain at all in the chest)
Typically at rest / Maybe brought on by Unusual Exercise / Argument / Intercourse / Snow shovelling etc.
Pain is prolonged / Often relieved only by opiate analgesia
Associated symptoms include SOB / Sweating / Nausea / Vomiting / Pallor / Greyness
Ask about any chest pain or SOB since admission.

PMH Ask about previous vascular disease
Angina – present in about 40%
Claudication
Cerebrovascular disease **(19)**
Hypertension / High Cholesterol / Diabetes

FH Particularly a history of ischaemic heart disease in first degree relative.

DH Prior to and since admission.
Was the patient put on a drip (thrombolysis)?
Is he now on aspirin?

ROS Chest pain / SOB / Swelling of calves

SH **Smoking habit** - before admission!
Employment may be profoundly affected e.g. HGV drivers banned if follow up exercise test abnormal after full thickness infarct.

EXAMINATION

General Appearance

Anaemia / Xanthomata / Xanthelasma / Corneal arcus / Tar staining / Pyrexia

CVS
Atrial fibrillation (**27**) (Common post MI)
Bradycardia (Heart block / Beta-blocker treatment)
BP often low post MI
Presence of 4th heart sound is very common
Look for signs of Left Ventricular Failure (**30**)
Poor cardiac output / Basal crackles / Dyspnoea
Evidence of peripheral vascular disease
Absent pulses / Femoral bruits / Carotid bruits

INVESTIGATIONS

Full Blood Count (FBC)
Erythrocyte Sedimentation Rate (ESR)
(Both White Cell Count (WCC) and ESR may be elevated)
Urea and Electrolytes (U&E) / Glucose
Cholesterol
Cardiac Enzymes (3 consecutive days)
Electrocardiogram (ECG)
Chest X-ray (CXR)

TREATMENT

Remember BOOMAR

B Bed rest
O Oxygen
O Opiate analgesia
M Monitor for arrhythmias
A Anticoagulate (subcutaneous heparin to prevent DVT)
R Reduce the size of the thrombus with streptokinase

Stop Smoking

COMPLICATIONS

Early Cardiac arrhythmias
Cardiac failure
Pericarditis
Recurrent infarction / Angina
Thrombo-embolism
Mitral regurgitation (Chordae rupture)
Ventricular septal / Free wall rupture

Late Cardiac failure **(30)**
Dressler's syndrome Weeks to months post MI / Autoimmune pericarditis / Fever / Pericardial effusion
Treatment NSAIDs / Steroids / Not anticoagulants
Ventricular aneurysm

Comment: Advice to give patient on discharge

Stop smoking
Review diet especially if overweight
Exercise Daily short walks **(x2)** *15–20 minutes duration*
Increase distance gradually
Avoid strenuous exercise
Avoid driving for 6 weeks
Sexual intercourse best avoided for 1 month
Most patients should aim to return to work 3 months later
Some of the occupations which may be affected
HGV/Public Service Vehicle driving
Airline piloting

CASE 2: INFECTIVE ENDOCARDITIS

An uncommon condition, but patients are usually in hospital for several weeks, and therefore appear relatively frequently in exams!

PC

Fever
Constitutional symptoms
Symptoms of cardiac failure **(30)** / Embolisation

HPC

Characteristically in infective endocarditis, at least in the sub-acute form, the symptoms are of such gradual onset that the patient often finds it impossible to date the onset of their illness.
Predisposing factors include previous dental and surgical procedures, so remember to ask specifically. The mean interval between the procedure and the diagnosis being made is 3 months.
Together with the fever there may be symptoms of sweats, chills or, rarely, rigors.
Symptoms of general malaise, anorexia, weight loss, aching joints etc. are often prominent – note their rather non-specific nature.
Occasionally the condition may present with complications secondary to embolisation e.g. stroke.

PMH

Around 50% are known to have pre-existing valve disease.
Ask for history of Rheumatic Fever / St. Vitus' Dance (Chorea)

EXAMINATION

General Appearance

Fever / Pallor / Evidence of weight loss
Petechial haemorrhages – Trunk / Limbs / Mucous membranes
Splinters / haemorrhages
Osler's nodes
Janeway lesions (looks like blotchy palmar erythema)
Roth spots (retinal haemorrhages with pale centre)
State of teeth / ? Dentures

CVS Tachycardia / Heart failure
Murmur – Most commonly aortic regurgitation or mitral regurgitation

Abdo Splenomegaly

Urinalysis
Microscopic haematuria and proteinuria

INVESTIGATIONS
Blood cultures x 6
Echocardiography to look for Vegetations / Valve damage
FBC – Mild normochromic, normocytic anaemia (Chronic Disease Picture)
ESR – Elevated
U&E

TREATMENT
Treatment of any underlying infection e.g. Dental abscess
Intravenous bactericidal antibiotics, according to results of Blood cultures
Surgery for extensive valvular damage / Prosthetic valve infection / Severe heart failure **(30)**

COMPLICATIONS
Embolisation (from the vegetations)
Stroke **(19)**
Renal infarction
Splenic infarction (splenic rub)
Osler's nodes
Immune complex formation
Glomerulonephritis (proteinuria)
Roth spots (retina)
Janeway lesions

Comment: Prosthetic valves

*Endocarditis on prosthetic valves **(29)** accounts for up to one-third of all cases. Early infection – within two months of surgery – carries a* *particularly high mortality. Established infection will cause alteration of the prosthetic valve sounds – 'muffling' them.*

Intravenous drug users are at risk of developing ***right-sided*** *endocarditis; usually the tricuspid valve is affected. Typically the patient is a young male, with no known history of heart disease and a fairly short history. In these cases embolisation commonly causes pulmonary infarction +/- abscess formation.*

CASE 3: BRONCHIAL CARCINOMA

PC **Chest symptoms** Worsening cough / Haemoptysis / Chest pain / Hoarse voice / Stridor / Breathlessness / Pneumonia

HPC **Other symptoms** Back pain / Bony pain / Headache (Metastatic) / Thirst / Polyuria / Leg weakness / Sensory disturbance / Lethargy

PMH History of: chronic bronchitis (in view of their common aetiologies) / TB / Pulmonary fibrosis (association with adenocarcinoma)

FH

ROS Ask about complications of the disease and its treatment.

SH **Smoking habit** / Passive smoking
Occupation: Asbestos / Chromium / Nickel exposure

EXAMINATION
General Appearance
Cachectic / Breathless / Muscle wasting

Hands Tar staining / Clubbing

Neck Lymphadenopathy **(55)**

Face Horner's **(61)** / Hoarse voice (recurrent laryngeal nerve palsy) / SVCO **(33)**

Resp Pleural effusion **(31)** / Lobar collapse / Consolidation / May be normal
Radiotherapy marks / Operation scars

Abdo Hepatomegaly / Ascites

CNS Papilloedema / Myopathy / Neuropathy / Cerebellar syndrome

Other There are many non-metastatic complications of malignancy especially with small (oat) cell carcinoma of the lung. You should be familiar with the commonest of these.

Cachexia / Weight loss
Hypercalcaemia / Hyponatraemia (SIADH) / Ectopic ACTH
Hypertrophic pulmonary osteoarthropathy (HPOA)
Clubbing
Polyneuropathy / Autonomic neuropathy / Polymyositis
Dermatomyositis / Lambert Eaton myasthenic syndrome / Cerebellar syndrome
Dementia / Myelopathy
Thrombophlebitis migrans / Anaemia / Polycythaemia
Acanthosis nigricans

INVESTIGATIONS

FBC
LFTS / Calcium / Sodium
CXR
Sputum cytology
Bronchoscopy / Pleural aspiration / Pleural biopsy
Pulmonary function tests (if contemplating surgery)
CT thorax
(USS abdomen / bone scan / CT brain)

TREATMENT

Surgery Suitable in 20%

Attention to Age
Lung function / Hilar and Mediastinal nodes
Metastatic disease / Cell type

RadioRx	Best for squamous cell carcinoma Used in those with 'operable' tumour not resected for other reasons Palliation for pain / Recurrent haemoptysis / Severe dyspnoea
ChemoRx	Reserved for small cell carcinoma

Comment: Three main histological types of bronchial tumour

Squamous	*Slow-growing / Metastasises late* *Associated with clubbing / HPOA / Hypercalaemia (due to PTHrP release)*
Small cell	*Fast-growing / Metastases usually present at the time of diagnosis* *Associated with SIADH / ectopic ACTH etc.*
Adenocarcinoma	*Proportionally more common in non-smokers*

CASE 4: CHRONIC BRONCHITIS AND EMPHYSEMA

PC Cough / Sputum / SOB / Wheeze

HPC History extending back over many years of cough productive of scanty mucoid sputum, esp. in mornings (regarded by many smokers as normal), accompanied by increasing shortness of breath and decreasing exercise tolerance.
Admission often precipitated by 'infective exacerbation': sputum turns green, increases in amount / SOB / fever etc.
Ask specifically about ankle swelling.

Smoking habit – Smoker / Ex-Smoker / Life long Non-Smoker (unlikely!)

FH If the patient is young (< 40) may be α_1 antitrypsin deficiency.

DH Inhaled / Nebulised bronchodilators (salbutamol / terbutaline)
Steroids
Home oxygen

SH Exercise tolerance when well. Are they able to leave the house, shop etc?

EXAMINATION

General Appearance

Dyspnoeic / Cyanosed / Febrile / Tar-stained fingers / Plethoric

CVS Cor Pulmonale: Raised JVP / Loud P2 / Ankle oedema (The parasternal heave is usually obliterated by hyperinflated lungs.)

Resp Tachypnoeic
Accessory muscles of respiration / Lip-pursing / Tracheal tug / Recession

Decreased expansion / Increased resonance of percussion note
Quiet breath sounds / Prolonged expiratory phase / Widespread wheezes

Abdo Liver often 'pushed down' by hyperinflated lungs.

INVESTIGATIONS

FBC (Polycythaemia secondary to chronic hypoxaemia)
CXR
Sputum microscopy / Culture / Sensitivity (MCS)
Pulmonary function tests (PEFR/ FEV_1/ FVC)
Arterial blood gases
ECG (looking for changes of right heart 'strain')

TREATMENT

Stop Smoking
Bronchodilators
Steroids (Only if a significant element of reversibility)
Antibiotics
Controlled oxygen therapy*
Physiotherapy for retained secretions

*It has been shown that long-term oxygen therapy (minimum 15 hours/day at 2 l/min) can reduce mortality in certain patients (those with: FEV_1<1.5l / PaO_2<7.3 kPa / Peripheral oedema).

Comment

Definitions: *Chronic bronchitis is a* ***clinical*** *definition – the production of sputum on most days for 3 months of the year in 2 consecutive years.*

Emphysema is a ***pathological*** *diagnosis – enlargement of air spaces distal to the terminal bronchiole, accompanied by destruction of their walls.*

It used to be popular practice to divide patients clinically into ***Blue Bloaters*** *(cyanosed and oedematous with stocky necks) and* ***Pink Puffers*** *(thin and breathless, but not cyanosed). The former were thought principally to suffer with chronic bronchitis and the latter with emphysema. However this clinical impression is not borne out by pathological studies, and in fact has more to do with differences in the sensitivity of the respiratory centre.*

CASE 5: CYSTIC FIBROSIS

PC	Presenting symptoms	Meconium ileus / Recurrent chest infections
HPC	Method of diagnosis	Sweat test / Lung function / GI absorption
	Chest	Breathless / Sputum / Haemoptysis / Wheeze / Infection Pneumothorax
	GI	Weight loss / Constipation / Cirrhosis (jaundice)
	Cardiac failure	Secondary to pulmonary hypertension / Heart-Lung transplant
	Diabetes 10%	
	General	Lethargy in hot weather due to salt loss
	Nasal polyps	
	Decreased fertility	95% azoospermia
	Who helps with Postural Drainage?	
	How many admissions to hospital?	
PMH		
Drugs		
FH	Autosomal recessive. Gene frequency 1:50 explains 60–70% positive FH.	
ROS	Go over any complications not mentioned during the PC.	
SH	Problems with schooling / Employment	

EXAMINATION

General Appearance

Short stature / Decreased muscle bulk with severe disease

Clubbing

Chest Cough (look at sputum) / Pneumothorax / Crackles / Wheeze

CVS Cor Pulmonale: Raised JVP / Ankle oedema / Right ventricular heave

GI Cirrhosis

INVESTIGATIONS

Sputum culture (*Haemophilus* / *Pseudomonas*)
Pulmonary function tests
CXR Increased lung markings / Consolidation / Pneumothorax
FBC Anaemia / Increased WCC with infection
U&E Salt loss / LFTs (? picture of Cirrhosis)

TREATMENT

Physiotherapy / Postural drainage
Drugs Pancreatic enzyme supplements / Inhalers / Vitamins
Heart-Lung transplant
Gene replacement (Experimental at this stage but a very important concept)

Comment

Life expectancy has gradually increased and the mean is now about 35 years.

CASE 6: CHRONIC LIVER DISEASE

PC Often non-specific: Lethargy / Anorexia / Nausea / Vague abdominal discomfort / Ankle swelling / Easy bruising / Pruritus / Jaundice

HPC Likely to have been non-specifically unwell for some time
Precipitating factors: Haematemesis / Infection / Operations
Previous admissions

PMH Previous episodes of jaundice
Blood transfusions / Intravenous drug use
Auto-immune diseases **(53)** (associated with Chronic Active Hepatitis, CAH)
Emphysema (α_1 antitrypsin deficiency)
Thrombotic tendency (Budd-Chiari)

FH Enquire carefully
It is crucial to identify treatable causes of CLD
E.g. Haemochromatosis / Wilson's disease

DH May be the cause e.g. Methyldopa / Nitrofurantoin (rare)
Phenothiazines cause cholestatic jaundice

ROS Amenorrhoea / Impotence / Loss of libido

SH TAKE A CAREFUL ALCOHOL HISTORY **(18)**
Remember high risk occupations: Licensing trade / Travelling salesmen / Doctors
Hepatitis risk IV Drug use / Sexuality

EXAMINATION

Most physical findings in CLD are given under the heading 'examine this patient's abdomen'. It is important to look carefully for any factors that will lead you to the underlying cause of the liver failure e.g. Hepatitis / Haemochromatosis / Wilson's disease / Alcohol excess / Tattoos.

The abdominal signs will usually involve **Hepatomegaly (35)** ± **Splenomegaly (36) / Ascites (38)** (in long standing cirrhosis the liver is small and shrunken but there will be evidence of portal hypertension). Abdominal scars may reflect Portal shunting / Variceal repair / Transplantation.

Indicators of decompensation

Encephalopathy (Decreased detoxification)
Oedema (Low albumin)
Ascites
Foetor
Flap / Tremor
Bruising (especially at needle sites)

INVESTIGATIONS

FBC High MCV
Low Platelets (Hypersplenism)
Prothrombin time
LFTs / Albumin
U&Es
Hepatitis screen (B and C)
ANA / SMA / AMA (Primary biliary cirrhosis PBC)
Immunoglobulins (IgA Alcohol / IgM PBC / IgG CAH)
Iron studies (Haemochromatosis)
Abdominal ultrasound / Gastroscopy (? varices)
Liver biopsy
α–fetoprotein (Hepatocellular carcinoma)
α_1 Antitrypsin level
Copper studies (Wilson's disease)

Comment

Chronic liver disease is the diagnosis you can make at the bedside; cirrhosis is a histological diagnosis, and is made on the results of a liver biopsy. Clotting problems are due to hypersplenism (low platelets) and the lack of liver-produced clotting factors (II, VII, IX, X). VII has the shortest half life hence the prothrombin time is the first to become abnormal.

***'Liver function'** may be assessed in terms of **Synthetic function** (Albumin / Clotting factors) and **Detoxification** (Encephalopathy).*

'Liver function tests' enable you to assess hepatocellular damage (high enzyme levels of AST / ALT) or Biliary obstruction (raised bilirubin / alkaline phosphatase).

CASE 7: INFLAMMATORY BOWEL DISEASE

PC

Crohn's disease — Diarrhoea / Abdominal pain / Weight loss / Malaise

Ulcerative colitis — Diarrhoea with blood and mucus / Abdominal pain

HPC Both diseases are relapsing / remitting in nature, and many patients enjoy good health most of the time. The patient in the exam, however, is more likely to have severe disease. Patients with extensive **Crohn's** may have had several surgical operations for intestinal obstruction secondary to Stricture formation / Fistulas / Failure of medical management. The patient with **Ulcerative colitis (UC)** may have been admitted to hospital for a severe attack of colitis with toxic megacolon. Occasionally surgery is needed (ileostomy and total colectomy).

PMH Ankylosing spondylitis

FH Increased familial incidence, but no clear-cut pattern of inheritance.

DH

ROS Dry, gritty red eyes / Arthralgia / Rashes

SH Crohn's more common in smokers
UC more common in non-smokers

EXAMINATION

General Appearance

Thin / Pale / Febrile
Erythema nodosum **(48)** / Arthropathy

Hands Finger clubbing **(43)** rarely

Face Conjunctivitis

Mouth Swollen lips / Aphthous ulcers

Abdo Multiple laparotomy scars / Fistulae / Thickened tender mass in RIF (Crohn's)
Distension / Tenderness (UC)

Note: You will NOT be expected to perform a rectal examination, but you should know what you might expect to find: Oedematous skin tags / Fissuring / Ulceration / Fistulae.

INVESTIGATIONS

FBC / ESR / C-reactive protein
Albumin
Liver function tests (Sclerosing cholangitis with UC)
Blood cultures
Stool cultures

Sigmoidoscopy (Rigid / Flexible) with Biopsies
Small Bowel Enema / Meal with Follow Through (Crohn's)
Barium Enema
Colonoscopy with Biopsies
Radiolabelled white cell scan (in severe disease when radiology and endoscopy contraindicated)

TREATMENT

Maintenance

Diet (Appropriate fibre intake)
5-ASA Compounds
Vitamins
Iron

Relapse

Mild: Steroids (Oral / Retention enemas)
Increase dose of 5-ASA drugs

Severe: Admit to hospital
Nil By Mouth
Intravenous Fluids / Steroids / Antibiotics (if Septic)
Daily Abdominal X-ray (Colonic disease)
Surgery
Parenteral nutrition
Severe and / or continually relapsing disease may respond to immunosuppressant drugs (azathioprine) or an elemental diet.

Comment: Examiners may expect you to know the pathology of the two diseases.

Crohn's *Affects any part of GI tract '**mouth to anus**' / Most frequently the terminal ileum*
Macro Thickened / Narrowed bowel / Cobblestone appearance / 'Skip' lesions
*Micro Inflammation involves ALL layers / **Granulomas***

UC *Extends proximally from the rectum (occasionally involves the terminal ileum – 'backwash ileitis')*
Macro Red, inflamed mucosa / Bleeds easily / Inflammatory polyps
*Micro Inflammation limited to the mucosa / **Crypt abscesses***

*REMEMBER – **UC and colonic Crohn's are potentially pre-malignant conditions.***

Both diseases have a wide range of extra-intestinal manifestations, some of which are related to disease activity. You should know about them.

CASE 8: RHEUMATOID ARTHRITIS

PC **Joint Pain** / **Swelling** / Stiffness
Fatigue / Malaise

HPC Which joints affected / **Symmetrical** pattern
Duration of 'Early Morning Stiffness'
Acute joint swelling (? Effusion)
Disability: Fasten buttons / Brush hair / Climb stairs / Walk etc.

Symptoms of extra-articular complications

Chest pain	Pericarditis
SOB	Pleural effusion / Fibrosing alveolitis / Anaemia
Dry eyes	Painful red eyes Sjögren's / Scleritis
Neurological	Nerve entrapment / Peripheral neuropathy
Skin	Raynaud's / Nodules / Ulceration

PMH Previous peptic ulceration (Care with NSAIDs)

DH List all treatment Past and Present
Was past treatment stopped due to side effects or lack of response?
Ask about joint injections (steroids)

FH Family history in 5–10%

ROS

SH In particular note the functional ability, consider helpful gadgets around the house and whether walking aids or a wheelchair are needed.

EXAMINATION

General Appearance

Pale / Tired / Unwell / Febrile / Leg ulcers / Lymphadenopathy

Hands (40)

All other joints must be examined for

Swelling   Synovitis / Effusion
Pain
Erythema
Limitation of movement

Face Dry eyes / Scleritis / Scleromalacia

CVS Pericardial rub

Resp Pleural effusion (**31**) / Fibrosis (lower zones)

Abdo Splenomegaly (Felty's syndrome)

CNS Carpal tunnel (**44**) / Peripheral neuropathy (**86**)

Urine Proteinuria (Drugs / Amyloid)

INVESTIGATIONS

FBC   Anaemia (Normochromic-Normocytic)
Thrombocytosis

ESR / PV   Elevated

Rheumatoid Factor (80%) Anti-nuclear antibody (30%)

Synovial fluid analysis

X-Rays   Soft tissue swelling / Narrowing of joint space
Erosions / Periarticular osteoporosis

TREATMENT

Drugs   You should know the most important side effects:

NSAIDs   Peptic ulcers / Iron deficiency anaemia secondary to blood loss

Sulphasalazine   Nausea / Headache / Marrow toxicity / Hepatitis / Oligospermia

Penicillamine   Metallic taste / Thrombocytopenia / Proteinuria (Nephrotic syndrome)

Gold   Rash / Thrombocytopenia / Proteinuria (Nephrotic syndrome)

Steroids   Weight gain / Osteoporosis / Cushing's (**92**)

Chloroquine	Retinopathy
Azathioprine	Nausea / Marrow toxicity / Infections e.g. Shingles (herpes zoster)
Methotrexate	Marrow toxicity / Pulmonary hypersensitivity / Hepatic fibrosis

Intra-articular steroids are used to manage acute exacerbations in one or two joints at a time. Joints should not be injected more than 2–3 times in any one year. Complications such as joint infection and skin ulceration may develop if given inappropriately or incorrectly.

Aids / Splints / Physiotherapy / General support

Comment

Rheumatoid arthritis is a common disease and appears as a long case frequently. The patient in the exam with RA may have been admitted for one of three reasons:

1. *Directly due to joint disease*
2. *Extra-articular disease*
3. *Complications of treatment*

Hence you need to be familiar with all these aspects of the disease.

Note: the hallmark of an inflammatory arthropathy is early morning stiffness – although this can occur in osteoarthritis it is usually of short duration (1/2 hour). Contrast the pattern of joint involvement in RA – Proximal Interphalangeal Joints (Proximal IPJs), Metacarpo-phalangeal Joints (MCPs), wrist, elbow, shoulder, knee, ankle – with that in osteoarthritis – Distal IPJs, lumbar spine, knees and hips.

CASE 9: SYSTEMIC LUPUS ERYTHEMATOSUS

A similar case to rheumatoid arthritis in its approach. The patients are usually young females and tend to be well informed about their condition – use their expertise!

PC Initial presentation: When / Precipitating event?

HPC SLE is extremely variable in its manifestation. **Arthralgia** and **Rash** are the commonest features, but it is a truly multi-system disorder and all the following must be enquired about. (Your systemic enquiry will be exhausted during this part of the history.)

General Weight loss / Malaise / Fever

Joints Pain / Swelling

Skin Facial rash / Photosensitivity / Raynaud's

Resp Pleuritic chest pain / Shortness of breath

Renal Treatment for renal failure / Dialysis

Neuro Fits / Stroke-like episodes

PMH Recurrent abortions (use 'miscarriages' with the patient)
Previous DVT / PE
History of Depression **(15)** / Psychosis **(16)**

FH

DH Rarely certain drugs can produce a SLE-like syndrome eg penicillamine

SH

EXAMINATION

General Appearance

Pallor / Pyrexia / Lymphadenopathy / Vasculitic rash

Hands Raynaud's / Nail bed infarcts / Finger spindling

Face Butterfly rash (Sun sensitive)

CVS Hypertension (related to renal disease)

Resp Pleural rub / Effusion **(31)**

B&J Often normal (despite severe pain) / Spindling of fingers
May have severe arthritis

Nerves Mononeuritis / Psychosis / Depression
Signs of previous CVA (Thrombotic) **(19)**

Urine **Proteinuria / Haematuria**

INVESTIGATIONS

FBC	Anaemia of chronic disease / Leucopenia
ESR	Elevated
U&E	Renal disease
ANA	95%
ds-DNA	50% (but specific)
Complement	Low in active disease
Rh. Factor	50%
(Renal biopsy)	

TREATMENT

Chloroquine Mild disease
Steroids The 'mainstay' of treatment
Cyclophosphamide / Azathioprine / Serious disease (renal or cerebral involvement)
Avoid sunlight / Use sun block if photosensitive

Comment

There is a distinct overlap between the connective tissue diseases and this often confuses candidates and examiners alike. Mixed Connective

Tissue Disease (MCTD) is a useful term for cases with features of more than one of SLE, Systemic sclerosis ***(45)*** *and Polymyositis* ***(47)****. Investigation shows antibodies to ribonucleoprotein (part of the extractable nuclear antigen, ENA) in a speckled pattern.*

CASE 10: CHRONIC RENAL FAILURE

Think of CRF as a multisystem disorder. Patients with CRF often spend long periods in hospital.

PC Reason for admission – New diagnosis / Dialysis problem / Complication

HPC When was renal failure first diagnosed, and what were the symptoms: lethargy, fatigue, anorexia, nausea, vomiting, pruritus.
May have been picked up because of the discovery of anaemia / hypertension.
Cause of renal failure? On dialysis? If so, how long?
Continuous Ambulatory Peritoneal Dialysis (CAPD)

	How many exchanges per day (Light bags / Heavy bags)
	How many episodes of CAPD – peritonitis
Haemodialysis	Hospital / Home
	Vascular access Arm / Neck / ? Problems
Transplant	Functioning / Failed

PMH Ask about disease responsible for causing renal failure if known
? Vascular disease: Angina / MI / TIAs / CVA / Claudication
Complications: Hypertension / Bone disease / Anaemia
Is patient aware of any problem with calcium metabolism? May be awaiting parathyroidectomy.

DH Likely to be taking several drugs: Anti-hypertensives / Vitamin supplements / Phosphate binders / Calcium salts Erythropoietin

FH Relevant for certain causes of renal failure
E.g. Polycystic kidneys **(39)** / Alport's Disease (Autosomal dominant + Sensorineural deafness)

SH Likely to be unable to work
Ask about invalidity benefit etc.
? Home alterations to facilitate home haemodialysis
If CAPD, does the patient have a separate room for the purpose?

EXAMINATION

General appearance

Anaemic / Pigmentation **(95)** / Excoriation (Pruritus) / Bruising
Look for A-V fistula (shunt) – usually the forearm
Neck dialysis lines / Scars from previous insertions

CVS Hypertension / Heaving apex beat / Loud 2nd heart sound

Abdo Polycystic kidneys / Transplanted kidneys
Tenckhoff catheter – check exit site clean and healthy

CNS Fundi – hypertensive retinopathy **(71)**
Peripheral neuropathy **(86)**

Urinalysis The patient is very likely to be anuric!

INVESTIGATIONS

FBC / U&E / Calcium / Phosphate / Alkaline phosphatase
Creatinine clearance / Ultrasound scan
Isotope renogram / Intravenous urography
Renal biopsy (difficult if the kidneys are small and shrunken)

TREATMENT

Diet. All patients with CRF will have been placed on a fairly strict 'renal' diet. The essential features are protein, potassium, phosphate and salt restriction. Foods which are restricted / excluded include chocolate, coffee, bananas, fruit drinks, dairy products.

Drugs. By the time end-stage renal failure (ESRF) occurs virtually all patients are hypertensive, whatever the cause of renal impairment, and will be on anti-hypertensives.

To prevent bone disease it is crucial to maintain normal plasma levels of phosphate and calcium: calcium carbonate is most frequently used (Calcichew), sometimes vitamin D.
The patient may require anti-histamines for pruritus, or anti-emetics for nausea.
Erythropoietin, by subcutaneous injection, is used to counteract the anaemia of CRF.

Dialysis. When the patient reaches ESRF dialysis is implemented, either with CAPD or haemodialysis.
CAPD is increasingly used. Typically the patient uses 4 exchanges per day, each of which is a 2 litre bag of dialysate fluid. The glucose content, and hence the osmolality, can be varied according to the need to remove fluid (the patient will be aware of his ideal 'dry' weight). The 'Achilles Heel' of CAPD is CAPD-peritonitis, which usually manifests itself initially as a 'cloudy bag'.
Insulin can be added to the dialysate fluid, for those with diabetes.

Haemodialysis usually involves 2–3 trips each week to hospital, each for around 6 hours. Some patients carry out their own haemodialysis at home. There may be problems with vascular access.

Transplantation. This requires less 'work' by the patient but involves long term immunosuppression which carries its own risks. Graft rejection remains a problem, as does the lack of available donor kidneys.

Comment

The common causes of CRF are:

Chronic glomerulonephritis
Chronic pyelonephritis
Diabetes mellitus (13)
Polycystic kidneys

CASE 11: NEPHROTIC SYNDROME

PC Swollen ankles / legs
Frothy urine

HPC The Nephrotic syndrome comprises the classical triad of **Proteinuria / Hypoalbuminaemia / Oedema** (many would add Hypercholesterolaemia).
Since three of these are essentially laboratory findings, oedema is the only major symptom. Heavy proteinuria can sometimes produce 'frothy urine'.
However, in less severe or very early cases, the disease may be picked up through 'asymptomatic' proteinuria or hyperlipidaemia.
Ask specifically about haematuria and preceding infections.

PMH RA / SLE / Diabetes
Known malignancy – Hodgkin's Lymphoma / Myeloma **(12)**
Tuberculosis / Osteomyelitis / Hepatitis B

FH Familial nephritides, especially Alport's

DH Take a careful drug history. Penicillamine / Gold (used in the treatment of RA **(8)**) and captopril (used in Hypertension / CCF **(30)**) are the chief culprits
Enquire specifically about a history of atopy.

ROS
SH

EXAMINATION
General Appearance

Face Facial / Peri-orbital oedema / Xanthelasma / Butterfly rash

CVS Hypertension
Signs of CCF

Resp Pleural effusions **(31)** if oedema very severe

Abdo May be Ascites **(38)** / Hepatosplenomegaly **(37)** / Other signs of chronic liver disease **(6)**

CNS ? Diabetic (**13**) / Hypertensive retinopathy (**71**)
Peripheral neuropathy (**86**) – may be a feature of DM / RA / SLE

Urinalysis
Heavy proteinuria (± haematuria)

INVESTIGATIONS
Urine microscopy
24 hour urinary protein / Creatinine clearance
U&E / Blood glucose / FBC (normochromic normocytic anaemia)
Albumin
Rh. Factor / ds-DNA / Anti-Neutrophil Cytoplasmic Antibody
Complement
Hepatitis B surface antigen
Serological tests for syphilis
Serum electrophoresis
CXR
Renal biopsy (unless child / long-standing Diabetes / drug-induced)

TREATMENT
Diuretics ± Fluid restriction
Salt restriction
Angiotensin Converting Enzyme (ACE) inhibitors (to reduce the protein leak)
Treat hypertension
Treat hypercholesterolaemia
Steroids for minimal change nephropathy and membranous nephropathy

Complication Renal vein thrombosis

Comment

*The causes of the Nephrotic syndrome can be divided into four main groups: The **Glomerulonephritides** and Minimal Change Nephropathy / **Drugs** / **Diabetes** / **Amyloid.***

CASE 12: MULTIPLE MYELOMA

PC Bone Pain
Lassitude
Infection

HPC Bone pain, and especially back pain, is by far the commonest presenting symptom: there may be an underlying pathological fracture.
Lassitude is a prominent feature, and indeed in some is the sole complaint.
Anorexia, vomiting and depression may all occur – secondary to hypercalcaemia.
Because the symptoms tend to be rather insidious and non-specific, they have often been present for some time before the diagnosis is made.
The varied nature of the symptoms means that the patient may present to many different specialties, e.g. orthopaedic surgeons, general physicians, haematologists, and for those patients who present with renal failure, nephrologists.
In 10% the presentation is with **infection**. Pneumonia is characteristic, especially Streptococcal.

PMH
FH No familial incidence
DH
ROS
SH

EXAMINATION
General Appearance
Pale / Tired / Unwell
May be in obvious pain secondary to pathological fracture
? Dehydrated / ? Uraemic
Easy bruising

CVS Very rarely heart failure secondary to hyperviscosity

Resp ? Pneumonia (Bronchial breathing / Crackles / Effusion etc.)

B&J Examine back (Erythema ab igne (**51**)) Vertebral collapse may cause loss of height

CNS Peripheral neuropathy can occur

INVESTIGATIONS

Diagnostic criteria – Need two or more of:
- Paraprotein in serum
- Bence-Jones protein in the urine
- Plasma cells in bone marrow

FBC (normochromic, normocytic anaemia)
ESR (elevated, often to over 100)
U&Es (impaired renal function)
Hypercalcaemia (with normal alkaline phosphatase cf. Bony Mets – Both up)
Skeletal Survey

TREATMENT

General measures	Analgesia / Rehydration
Specific	Chemotherapy / Dialysis

Comment

Multiple myeloma can affect many organ systems. The major effects of the disease can be divided into four groups:

The abnormal paraprotein itself
Hyperviscosity (raised ESR) / Abnormal platelet function / ***Renal damage*** */ Amyloid deposition*
Infiltration of the bone marrow
Anaemia */ Leucopenia / Thrombocytopenia*
Suppression of normal immunoglobulin
Poor humoral immunity and repeated infections
Skeletal Destruction
Pathological fracture / Vertebral collapse / ***Hypercalcaemia*** */* ***Pain***

CASE 13: DIABETES MELLITUS

Patients are frequently in hospital, either for treatment of their diabetes itself or, more commonly, for treatment of its complications.

PC **Polyuria / Thirst / Weight loss** (Insulin dependent)
Complications if longer standing (Non Insulin dependent presentation)

Retinopathy	Poor acuity / Blindness / Cataracts
Nephropathy	Hypertension
Neuropathy	Polyneuropathy – Sensory problems / Pain Mononeuropathy – Femoral amyotrophy / Carpal tunnel Autonomic neuropathy / Impotence / Diarrhoea etc
Vascular disease	Peripheral / Cardiovascular / Cerebrovascular

HPC When diagnosed / Who by / How
How does patient monitor diabetes: BM stix / Urinalysis
How good is control
What treatments so far (See below)
Symptoms of moniliasis
Necrobiosis lipoidica **(50)**

PMH May be extensive
Hypertensive

FH Increased risk in relatives

DH Diet / Oral hypoglycaemics
Insulin Which type: Pig / Human
Short / Long acting (or mixture)
Dose / Timing
Sites of injection (? lipohypertrophy)
Hypoglycaemic attacks

ROS Concentrate on complications not mentioned above

SH

EXAMINATION

General Appearance

Well / Unwell
Thin / Obese

CVS Particularly BP
Check foot pulses

Abdo Injection sites

CNS Visual acuity / Funduscopy **(70)**
Peripheral neuropathy **(86)**
Absent ankle jerks / Distal sensory loss / Neuropathic ulcers

The diabetic foot

Peripheral pulses
Skin Ulcers / Callous / Fungal infection / Nail care
Neuropathy

INVESTIGATIONS

For the patient in the exam, who is likely either to have had diabetes for many years or to have presented in diabetic ketoacidosis, the diagnosis is unlikely to be in doubt. However you should be aware of the strict diagnostic criteria.

Glycosylated haemoglobin (HbA_{1c})
U&E
Cholesterol

TREATMENT

Diet – ALL patients. The diet for a diabetic is no different from the diet considered healthy for the population as a whole.
Oral hypoglycaemics
Insulin   Human v Porcine
    Short / Intermediate / Long-acting

Comment

Essentially there are two types of diabetes:

Insulin dependent diabetes mellitus (IDDM / Type 1)

Young patient / Thin
Short history / Often presents in Ketoacidosis (DKA)
Treated with insulin from time of diagnosis

Non-insulin dependent diabetes mellitus (NIDDM / Maturity onset / Type 2)

Middle-aged / Overweight
Often been present 'subclinically' for some time, as the degree of hyperglycaemia is usually less, and hence often presents with complications of diabetes rather than thirst, weight loss etc.
Treated with diet alone / Oral hypoglycaemics / Occasionally insulin later.

CASE 14: HYPERTHYROIDISM / GRAVES' DISEASE

A common disorder, and although patients are often managed as outpatients, the symptoms and signs are so classical that they often appear in medical finals.

PC Varied
Typically – Weight loss / Palpitations / Anxiety / SOB

HPC Symptoms may have been present for some time before the diagnosis is made, as they are very variable, and often non-specific. Indeed many patients are often initially given a 'psychiatric' label.
Ask specifically about Heat intolerance / Diarrhoea / Goitre / Change in appearance.

PMH There may be a history of other auto-immune disorders **(53)**

FH Frequently positive for Thyroid dysfunction / Other auto-immune disorders

DH Is patient on treatment already Beta-blockers / Carbimazole

ROS
SH

EXAMINATION
General Appearance
Thin / Nervous / Fidgety

Hands Sweaty palms / Tremor of the outstretched arms / Palmar erythema
Thyroid acropachy **(43)**

Neck Goitre / ? Bruit **(54)**

Face Exophthalmos / Lid retraction / Lid lag
Eyes **(68)**

CVS Tachycardia / Atrial fibrillation **(27)** / Bounding pulse
Signs of heart failure (especially in the elderly)

CNS Proximal muscle weakness **(87)**

Extra Look for pretibial myxoedema **(49)**

INVESTIGATIONS

Thyroid function tests (high free T4, T3 / Low TSH)
Imaging techniques if goitre very large and considering surgery
Radioisotope studies if solitary nodule

TREATMENT

Drugs Carbimazole* for the disease
Propranolol for the symptoms
Radio-active iodine (most patients eventually become hypothyroid)
Surgery indications: Large goitre / Toxic nodule

Causes of hyperthyroidism

Graves' disease - commonest
Solitary toxic nodule (Plummer's disease – about 5%)
Toxic multinodular goitre (especially the elderly)

* Agranulocytosis can rarely occur as a side-effect (idiosyncratic) of carbimazole. Patients should be told to immediately report sore throat, fever etc. and have their blood count checked every few weeks during initial treatment.

Comment

You need to distinguish those signs due to hyperthyroidism itself (i.e. simply due to an excess of circulating T3 and T4) from those signs which occur only in Graves' disease.

Hyperthyroidism	***Graves'***
Lid lag / Lid retraction	*Exophthalmos*
Tachycardia / AF	*Pretibial myxoedema*
High output state	*Acropachy*
Tremor	
Palmar erythema	
Proximal myopathy	

PSYCHIATRY: LONG CASE PLAN

There is no fundamental difference between the approach to a psychiatric long case and the approach to any other medical case. The length and detail of the history is greater and the mental state examination takes over from the physical examination in level of importance. However, you must be sure to exclude organic disease that may lead to psychiatric disturbance, e.g. SLE – Psychosis, Thyroid disease – Depression, and look for physical complications of psychiatric disease e.g. Chronic Liver Disease in alcoholism, Movement Disorders with psychotropic drugs.

Your overall aim is to produce a formulation that includes the differential diagnosis:

Organic psychoses
Functional psychoses
Non-psychotic disorders
Personality disorders

and its aetiology:

Predisposing factors
Precipitating factors
Maintaining factors

You should also be able to comment on appropriate investigations, treatments and the prognosis.

Introduce yourself and establish a rapport. (Some centres actually watch this part of the interview and mark you on your ability to establish rapport, and on your questioning style and ability to define the problem). It is hard to be relaxed under scrutiny but telling the patient that you are nervous because of the importance of the exam and that you feel as if you are taking your driving test again may help break the ice!

On starting questioning make good eye contact. Using some open questions such as “would you please tell me what has been going on in your life recently”, “tell me more”, “go on” should start the ball rolling. Use closed questions e.g. "how is your appetite" to define more detailed points.

PC In detail, use the patient's own words.

HPC Describe the development of symptoms and ask about any associated symptoms. Note the duration of the illness and how it was diagnosed.

PMH / P Psych.H

It is important to note any previous episodes of the same or similar symptoms as the presenting complaint (you may be the first to recognise a crisis in the patient's past that may have been psychotic or depressive).

FH Commonly positive for psychiatric disease

Personal history

Childhood
School
Sexual development
Marriages / Children
Occupation (Present and past)
Forensic (Convictions / Trouble with police)
Social history (as all long case histories)

Pre Morbid Personality

Interests / Relationships / Previous level of function
Coping skills

Drugs Prescribed and recreational

Smoking

Alcohol Number of units (more detailed if drug dependence)

Revision of general symptoms

Mental state examination

Behaviour / Appearance
Dress / Conscious level / Posture / Involuntary movements / Self care / Eye contact / Rapport

Speech
Speed / Quantity / Quality

Mood
Subjective / Objective / Variability / Autonomic activity (Sweaty etc)

Thought form and content
Abnormal beliefs / Suicidal / Preoccupations

Perception
Illusions / Hallucinations / Passivity
Depersonalisation

Orientation
Time / Person / Place

Attention and Concentration
Months / Days backwards / Serial 7s

Short-term memory
Address / Digit Span

Longer term memory
Prime minister etc. / Past life (above)

Abstraction
Difference between dwarf and boy / Proverbs

Insight
Do they realise they are ill / Are they willing to be treated

General examination

All systems as in any case

Investigations

Psychosocial
Medical

Treatments

Psychological
Physical / Medical

CASE 15: DEPRESSION

In the exam the patient is likely to know if they have this diagnosis and with luck they will tell you at the start.

PC Find out what the first symptoms were and when they happened.

HPC

Emotional Sad / Helpless / Anxious / Agitated

Cognitive Self dislike / Blame / Indecisiveness / Worthlessness / Hopelessness / Poor thinking / Suicide

Biological Sleep – Poor with early morning wakening
Appetite – Down (or up) / Weight – Down (or up)
Libido / Energy / Concentration (all decreased)
New symptoms – Headache / Backache / Dizziness etc.
Diurnal variation (worse in morning)

Precipitating Factors
Losses: Bereavement / Job / Divorce / Separation / Health / Other life events (usually stressful)

PMH Depression / Mania / Psychosis / Serious medical illness

FH Bipolar illness / Current illnesses (son with leukaemia etc.)

Personal History

Childhood losses / Insecurity / Abuse

Marriages — Divorce / Separation

Occupation — Job loss / Stress at work / Length of unemployment

Social — Money problems / Housing problems
Friends / Interests

Pre-morbid

Low self-esteem / Level of function / Coping skills / Locus of control

Drugs Treatment / Predisposing e.g. Beta blockers / Steroids / Anti-arrhythmics

Smoking

Alcohol May be excessive

ROS ? Thyroid or other general disorders

Mental State

Behaviour	Poor eye contact / Poor posture / Increased or Decreased activity / Self neglect
Speech	Slow / Little spontaneous / Coherent
Mood	Low
Thought	**Worthless / Hopeless / Guilt / Blame / Suicide**
Perception	May have hallucinations / Nihilistic delusions
Orientation	Usually normal
Memory	Impaired if attention down
Insight	May be preserved

EXAMINATION

General Appearance

Look for general medical illness

INVESTIGATIONS

Exclude organic disease
FBC / ESR / U&E / Calcium / TFT
ECG if palpitations

TREATMENT

If suicidal may need to "section" under Mental Health Act

Drugs Re-uptake inhibitors

Tricyclics	Imipramine / Clomipramine	
	Prothiaden / Lofepramine /	
	Amitriptyline	
Serotonin	Fluoxetine / Paroxetine	

Monoamine oxidase inhibitors (second line)
Phenelzine (old)
Moclobemide (new)

Electroconvulsive treatment if psychotic depression
Psychological treatment (cognitive therapy)

Comment

Often patients with an anxiety neurosis develop depression and features of both conditions coexist. During the history you must look for symptoms for anxiety e.g.

Palpitations	***Tachycardia***	***Bowel disturbance***	***Sweating***
Irritability	***Muscle pain***	***Swallowing problems***	***Phobias***
Panic attacks	***Agoraphobia***	***Pins and needles***	***Dizziness***

Be sure to elucidate any thyroid or cardiac disease and check whether the patient is using beta-agonist inhalers. Phaeochromocytoma is very rare. Treatment involves anxiety management and antidepressant drugs.

CASE 16: PSYCHOSIS / SCHIZOPHRENIA

PC "What has been going on in your life recently?"

HPC Prodromal phase — Loss of interest / Poor hygiene / Change in mood / Decline in function

The interview should find out whether there are any of the diagnostic features of schizophrenia (see teaching points) and also exclude mania, depression, intoxication and organic brain syndromes including epilepsy.

Look for precipitating factors / Recent life events

PMH Previous episodes of psychiatric disease
Deafness / Blindness (in elderly)

FH Positive family history is common

Personal Birth trauma
Erratic performance at school, especially boys.
Unable to have long term relationship
Poor employment record
Criminal record
Low income etc.
Poor housing / Living rough

Premorbid
Schizoid / Schizotypical personality / Withdrawn / Eccentric / Paranoid

Drugs Treatment ?depot injections
Cannabis / Amphetamines precipitate psychotic illness
Prescribed medication e.g. Intravenous steroids

Smoking

Alcohol May be excessive

ROS ? Epilepsy / Headaches (brain tumour) / Alcohol withdrawal

Mental State

Behaviour	Self neglect / Abnormal movements (treatment effects)
Speech	Varied / Incomprehensible / Neologisms
Mood	Blunted affect / Inappropriate affect (excess laughing etc.)
Thought	Insertion / Withdrawal / Broadcasting / Abnormal beliefs (? Jesus Christ) / In contact with TV set
Perception	Auditory hallucinations third person / Thought echo / Running commentary / Passivity feelings
Orientation	? Jesus Christ / In contact with TV set / Often normal
Attention	Often poor
Memory	Decreased if concentration poor
Insight	Depends on degree of treatment

Note: Some forms of schizophrenia have more negative features: Poverty of speech / Slow thought etc.

EXAMINATION

General Appearance

Signs of drug use / Brain tumour

INVESTIGATIONS

Psychosocial investigations

Drug screen / EEG / CT scan

TREATMENT

Drugs	Acute	Neuroleptic drugs e.g. chlorpromazine
	Chronic	Oral / Depot e.g. flupenthixol

Supportive

Decreased stress in the environment

Decreased expressed emotion in family

Rehabilitation

Day care

Comment

The diagnosis of schizophrenia is indicated by one or more of the following symptoms:

Disorders of thought possession

Thought insertion
Thought withdrawal
Thought broadcasting

Auditory hallucinations in which the person hears:

His own thoughts out loud (thought echo)
People discussing him in the third person
Voices forming a running commentary

Passivity feelings

Feeling under control of an outside influence

Delusions

Persistent delusions culturally / physically impossible
Delusional perception

Or two or more of the following:

Persistent hallucinations
Incoherent / Irrelevant speech / Mannerisms / Neologisms
Catatonic phenomena
Negative symptoms

For further details of this and other psychiatric diseases we would suggest Psychiatry in Medical Practice: Second Edition. *Goldberg, Benjamin and Creed. Routledge, London.*

CASE 17: ANOREXIA NERVOSA

PC When was the condition first brought to medical attention? Why?

HPC Fat in past
How has patient dieted or controlled calories
Ask about exercise (usually excessive)
Previous investigations for diarrhoea / metabolic problems / amenorrhoea
Ask about body image / fear of fatness
Bulimic episodes
Menstrual history

PMH Diabetes / Thyroid disease

FH Increased eating disorders in family members

Personal Disturbed family relationships
Avoidance of maturity including sexual relationships
Denial of family problems
Parental discord (Divorce / Separation)

Drugs Laxatives / Diuretics

Smoking
Alcohol
ROS Raynaud's phenomenon is common
Excess hair (lanugo) on face and back
Feel cold
Exclude differential conditions:
Diabetes
Weight loss – Hyperthyroidism / Inflammatory bowel disease
Amenorrhoea – **Ovarian / Pituitary disease**

Mental State

Behaviour	Normal
Speech	Normal

Mood Anxious / Depressed / Unconcerned about health
Thought Abnormal body image / May be Suicidal
Perception
Orientation
Attention
Memory
Insight Lacking re. Health

EXAMINATION

General Appearance

Thin / Cold peripheries / Lanugo hair
Ask for weight and height and calculate body mass index (weight in Kg divided by height in metres squared)
Note the absence of hyperthyroidism etc.

INVESTIGATIONS

Social investigation of family relationships
Glucose / Thyroid function tests
U&E (low K^+ with purgatives or diuretics)
Low serum protein / FSH, LH decreased / ACTH increased (stress response)

TREATMENT

Restore body weight
Behavioural programme, progressive introduction of rewards for weight gain
Psychotherapy Family therapy for younger patients
Individual therapy if older
May need to move away from family situation (Inpatient / Other carer)
May need antidepressant medication

OTHER COMMON PSYCHIATRIC LONG CASES

As part of your revision you may wish to make up similar long case plans for the other common cases:

Mania / Anxiety / Obsessive compulsive disorders / Personality disorder / Dementia / Korsakov's syndrome

CASE 18: SUBSTANCE ABUSE

This may relate to any drug but more often than not it applies to alcohol in which case there is an overlap with chronic liver disease. There develops a **compulsion** to use the drug, **increased tolerance** and **withdrawal symptoms** on stopping. You must look out for physical, psychological and social complications e.g. chronic liver disease, changes in mood, convictions and marriage breakdown and salience or stereotyped behaviour.

PC When first brought to medical attention?
Why?

HPC When first took the drug and when became used regularly or more heavily (?Amount)
Why did they first use the drug? Peer pressure / Anxiety / Depression / Availability
What effects did and does the drug have?
When first had problems with the drug / What problems?
How do they obtain (and pay for) the drug / How do they use it (Inject / Smoke etc)?
How has tolerance developed?
What withdrawal effects are noticed? Fits / Delirium Tremens / Cold turkey / Anxiety
What other symptoms of dependence?

PMH Depression or other psychiatric history
Chronic illness or chronic pain

FH Increased addictive behaviour in family members

Personal Childhood exposure to addictive behaviour / Abuse / Neglected childhood
Poor performance at school if glue sniffer
Poor employment record / **High risk occupation** (Barman / Traveller)
Criminal record: Theft / Violence / Drink Driving / Prostitution
Poor marital history (Divorce / Aggression)
Poor standard of living as money goes on drug habit

Premorbid

Drugs Any medication

Smoking Signs of addictive behaviour

Alcohol Number of units per week / Typical drinking day
The **CAGE** questionnaire indicates excessive drinking if there are two or more yes answers.

- **C** Have you ever felt you ought to **Cut** down on your drinking?
- **A** Have people **Annoyed** you by criticizing your drinking?
- **G** Have you ever felt **Guilty** about your drinking?
- **E** Have you ever had a drink first thing in the morning to steady your nerves or get rid of a hangover (**Eye opener**)?

ROS Here you must identify any associations with the particular drug. Chronic liver disease with alcohol and AIDS with iv drug use etc.
Chest infections / Cardiomyopathy / Endocarditis with iv drug abuse
Gastritis / Oesophagitis / Pancreatitis / Hepatitis
Stroke / Neuropathy / Cerebellar degeneration / Myopathy / Head injury / Korsakov's / Wernicke's syndromes with alcohol

Mental State

- **Behaviour** Poor self-care / Abnormal movements / Withdrawal symptoms
- **Speech** Cerebellar / Slurred
- **Mood** Anxiety / Depression
- **Thought** Suicide / Preoccupation with drugs / Paranoid ideas
- **Perception**
- **Orientation** Abnormal if intoxicated (Hopefully not during exam!)
- **Attention** Poor

Memory	Korsakov's – Poor retrograde memory
Insight	"I can kick it"; but they can't

EXAMINATION

General Appearance

Signs of the complications of the substance used
Needle marks / Phlebitis
AIDS
Chronic liver disease

INVESTIGATIONS

FBC, U&E, LFT and others depending on type of drug
Social investigations

TREATMENT

Acute	Treatment of withdrawal	
	Alcohol	Chlordiazepoxide regimen
	Opiates	Symptomatic / Methadone
Long term	Psychological support / Alcoholics Anonymous	
	Antabuse	
	Methadone	

Other treatment of underlying mood disorder

Comments

*The drugs most often abused are: **Alcohol / Opiates / Hallucinogens / Amphetamines / Cannabis / Solvents**. There may be a history of abuse of several drugs over the course of the illness and each of these should be mentioned.*

CASE 19: STROKE

PC	Weakness / Collapse / Visual disturbance / Dizziness / Speech problems / Sensory upset / Headache	
HPC	**Onset**	**Sudden**
	Course	Static / Resolving
	History	Previous CVA / TIAs Amaurosis Fugax Transient Sensory / Motor problems
	Risk factors	**Smoking** **Hypertension** **Diabetes** **Hyperlipidaemia**
	Right or left-handed?	
PMH	Angina / Myocardial infarction / Rheumatic heart disease (Atrial fibrillation) Claudication	
FH	Increased vascular disease in family members	
DH	Anti-hypertensive medication Aspirin Warfarin (may be the cause if haemorrhagic stroke)	
ROS	Ask about complications	
		Weight loss / Constipation / Bladder symptoms Shoulder subluxation / Pneumonia (Aspiration)
SH	Home	House type / Ground floor / Modifications (Stair lift / Bath seat / Downstairs commode)
	Dependants / Carers (Relatives / Friends / Home helps etc) Allowances	
	Mobility	Chair / Sticks / Zimmer

EXAMINATION

General Appearance

Plethoric / Malar flush

CVS Atrial fibrillation **(27)** / Heart murmurs
BP and signs of hypertensive heart disease
Carotid bruits

CNS Dysphasia **(82)** / Dysarthria / Apraxia / Sensory / Visual inattention

Cranials Homonymous hemianopia **(57)**
Facial weakness (UMN) **(76)**
Pseudobulbar palsy **(81)**

Limbs Hemiparesis UMN signs on one side +/- sensory loss

INVESTIGATIONS

FBC (Polycythaemia) / ESR
Glucose
ECG
CXR
Cholesterol
CT brain
Carotid Doppler ultrasound (even if no carotid bruits)
Echocardiogram if murmur

TREATMENT

Acute	Keep hydrated / Good nursing care / Do not treat initial hypertension
In-patient	Screen for risk factors / Nutrition / Aspirin Physiotherapy / Occupational therapy

---

Comment

Definition: a stroke is a sudden neurological deficit of vascular origin lasting longer than 24 hours.

Case 19: Stroke

Causes *Haemorrhage 15%*
(Subarachnoid haemorrhage 5% / Intracerebral 10%)
Infarction 85%
(Thrombotic / Embolic (from the heart or great vessels)

Clinical divisions

Carotid circulation	*Hemiparesis* *Homonymous Hemianopia* *Dysphasia / Neglect* *Hemisensory loss*
Vertebrobasilar	*Ipsilateral cranial nerve lesion / Contralateral Hemiparesis* *Cerebellar / Brainstem strokes*

CASE 20: MULTIPLE SCLEROSIS

The patient is often young.

PC Details of reasons for present admission e.g. difficulty walking, loss of balance, double vision, bladder symptoms, respite.

HPC When and how did patient first present
Course of illness to date – **Relapsing / Remitting v Chronic progressive**
If relapsing Number / Frequency / Nature of relapses
Ascertain level of patient's disability, if any, in their 'steady state'
Enquire carefully about bladder symptoms: Urgency / Urge incontinence
Recurrent UTIs
? Intermittent self-catheterisation / Urosheath / Indwelling catheter
It may be appropriate to ask male patients about impotence
Fatigue is very common

PMH

FH No clear cut pattern of inheritance: 5–15 x risk if first degree relative affected

DH Baclofen for spasticity / Anticholinergics for urge incontinence
IV steroids for recent relapse

ROS

SH This section of the history needs to be very thorough
Able to work / Invalidity benefit / Other allowance
Ambulant / Wheelchair / Able to transfer
Carer / District nurses / Home help

EXAMINATION

MS, by its very nature, can produce very varied clinical pictures: the following is an example.

General Appearance
Depressed / Euphoric / Anxious
The general examination is usually normal

CNS Cerebellar dysarthria (staccato speech)

Cranials Bilateral optic disc pallor **(72)**
Nystagmus **(64)** / Internuclear ophthalmoplegia **(65)** may be bilateral

Limbs Spasticity legs > arms / Clonus
Pyramidal weakness legs > arms **(85)**
All **reflexes very brisk** / Finger flexion jerks / Hoffman's present
Absent abdominal reflexes
Bilateral extensor plantars (very easy to elicit)
Sensation is often disturbed in a patchy distribution: any modality may be affected
Finger-nose ataxia in arms **(90)**
Gait – spastic and ataxic **(91)**

INVESTIGATIONS

Visual evoked responses (delayed-slow conduction in central white matter)

CSF 30% slight increase in mononuclear cells
40% slight increase in protein concentration
90% will have oligoclonal bands

MR imaging (High Signal lesions esp. periventricular)

TREATMENT

In acute relapses i.v. steroids have been shown to speed up the rate of recovery – although the *level* of recovery is unaltered. As yet there is no treatment available which has been conclusively shown to alter the course of the disease. Interferons may work.

Prognosis

Favourable	Onset:	Sensory symptoms / Optic neuritis (esp. if young)
Adverse	Onset:	Progressive course / Incomplete recovery from the initial attack Cerebellar ataxia / Persistent weakness

---

Comment

By definition the patient with multiple sclerosis must have a minimum of two episodes (lesions) separated both in time and place (position within the CNS). The course of MS is very variable: some patients have a gap of many years between relapses, others frequent relapses, and in others the disease runs a relentlessly progressive course from the outset.

The disease affects the white matter of the CNS causing ***demyelination*** *and has a predilection for the Optic nerves / Brainstem / Periventricular areas / Spinal cord.*
N.B. There is ***not*** *demyelination of the peripheral nerve.*

Involvement of the optic nerves causes ***optic or retrobulbar neuritis****. The characteristic clinical picture is that of unilateral visual loss over hours to days associated with pain, especially on moving the eye. Colour vision is particularly affected. Recovery is the rule. In optic neuritis nerve head swelling is seen (looks like papilloedema), in retrobulbar neuritis nothing is seen (the patient sees nothing, the doctor sees nothing).*

There are two unusual but very characteristic symptoms of MS. ***Uhthoff's phenomenon****: the effect of heat and exertion in temporarily increasing symptoms, most noticeably weakness of the legs and visual loss. The classic description is of being unable to get out of a hot bath.*

Lhermitte's sign *(really a symptom): electric-shock like sensations down the back, and sometimes the thighs on bending the neck. (Can occur in other diseases which involve the cervical spinal cord.)*

INTRODUCTION TO THE SHORT CASE

You will be taken to see a number of patients and given various instructions. Two examiners will take you, usually for about 30 minutes in which time you may see 4–6 cases. The types of case will usually be balanced between the systems; it would be unusual for a candidate not to be asked to examine the cardiovascular system.

You will be assessed on:

Your approach to the patient
Your ability to perform a careful competent examination
Your ability to pick up important signs
Your ability to interpret these signs

Your approach to the examiners is not formally tested but if good can only help in their overall assessment of you.

It is VERY important that you are polite to the patients, ask their permission to examine them and do not hurt them.

Approach to the patient

A good start may sound like this:
Examiner: *"Please examine this man's heart."*
Candidate, to patient (Make good eye contact with the patient and shake their hand): *"How do you do sir? I am Mr Smith. Would you mind if I examined your heart?"*
Patient: *"No."*
Candidate: *"Please would you take off your top and lean back on the pillows . . . Are you comfortable?* (Observe face etc.) *May I feel your pulse?"*

Approach to the examiners

On first meeting them make sure you introduce yourself. Try to answer the question asked and not something else!

During your short cases you may be encouraged to keep up a running commentary. If you have never done this before, practice it now. You may be allowed to continue uninterrupted but more often than not you will be stopped and started. This can be frustrating, but if you are prepared for it you should not allow it to disrupt your examination routine.

When you have finished examining the patient, thank them, make sure they are covered and then turn fully to face the examiners, try not to look away from them. Good eye contact and body posture help to present a competent appearance. Look at the spot at the top of the examiners nose and let rip! *"On examining Mr Smith's cardiovascular system, I have found evidence of mitral regurgitation without mitral stenosis that is not complicated by heart failure or infective endocarditis. This is evidenced by . . ."*

If you are not so sure about the diagnosis try: ***"I am uncertain about the definitive diagnosis but my differential diagnosis*** *is that of an ejection systolic murmur. Aortic stenosis is unlikely as the pulse character is normal, mitral regurgitation may be present but there is no radiation to the axilla. The other possibility is aortic sclerosis which is common in a man of this age".*

Each short case included in this book gives the main clinical features that may be present and some of the associated findings. We feel those cases included are the most common conditions seen in exams. We will have missed some cases that you or your teachers think relevant, however, if you are familiar with all these cases you should have little trouble in picking up most of the important features during the exam.

The **Teaching Points** and **Comments** give some associated and hopefully relevant facts. Many of these facts will be needed to answer extra questions during the clinical and also those asked during the viva-voce examination.

SHORT CASE INDEX

CARDIOVASCULAR SYSTEM
"Examine this Patient's Heart"

Introduce and Expose

Patient comfortable reclining at 45 degrees

Observe	Pallor	
	Dyspnoea	
	Cyanosis	
Hands	Clubbing **(43)**	
	Splinter Haemorrhages	Endocarditis
	Peripheral cyanosis	
	Cool peripheries	
	Tendon xanthomata	Hyperlipidaemia
	Tar staining	
Pulse (radial)	Rate	
	Rhythm	
	Radio-femoral delay in young adults (Coarctation of the aorta)	
	Check specifically for collapsing pulse **(24)**	
Blood pressure	Tell the examiner *"At this stage I would usually measure the blood pressure"*. If you are lucky you will be told what it is.	

Neck

Carotid pulse		Volume / Character / Thrill
JVP	Height	↑ + pulsatile in Right heart failure
		↑ + non-pulsatile in SVCO **(33)**
	Waveform	Giant systolic *V* waves in TR **(56)**
		May displace ear lobes

Face

Anaemia
Xanthelasma
Corneal arcus
Malar flush

With Patient Sitting Back

Praecordium

Inspect

Scars Median sternotomy (CABG / Valve replacement)
Lateral thoracotomy (Mitral valvotomy)
Apex visible

Palpate

Localise apex beat

Tapping	Palpable valve closure
Heaving	Sustained contraction
Thrusting	Hyperdynamic contraction

Thrills and parasternal heave

Percuss

Not usually performed

Auscultate

1. At apex with bell
2. Turn patient onto left hand side
   Relocate apex and listen specifically for Mitral Stenosis **(21)** (Held expiration)
   Turn patient back
3. At apex with diaphragm
   If murmur listen for radiation into axilla
4. Listen in all other areas
   Left sternal edge
   Pulmonary
   Aortic
5. Listen to Carotids (If no aortic murmur ? isolated carotid bruit)

Sit patient forward

Praecordium Listen specifically for the early diastolic murmur of aortic regurgitation (**24**) at left sternal edge in held expiration.

Lungs Listen at lung bases for inspiratory crackles

Sacrum Feel for sacral oedema whilst asking the patient *"does this hurt?"* This has the dual purpose of waking the examiner up and drawing attention to the fact you have looked for sacral oedema.

Feel for ankle oedema

Tell the examiner "To finish my examination I would like to see the temperature chart and dip the urine" (? Endocarditis).

When presenting your findings comment on the valve lesion(s) and whether it is complicated by heart failure or endocarditis. E.g. *"This lady has mitral stenosis, as evidenced by the mid-diastolic murmur heard loudest at the apex in held expiration, which is complicated by atrial fibrillation but not heart failure or endocarditis".*

Comment

Left sided murmurs increase in held expiration, right sided with inspiration.

CASE 21: MITRAL STENOSIS

Introduce and expose

Observe	? Female
Hands	
Pulse	**Atrial fibrillation (27)**
BP	Low with normal pulse pressure
Neck	JVP may be increased
	Giant V waves
Face	**Malar flush** (Cyanosis and telangiectasia)
Praecordium	
Inspect	? Left thoracotomy scar (Mitral valvotomy)
Palpate	**Undisplaced tapping** apex beat
	? Parasternal heave
Auscultate	**Loud 1st heart sound**
	Opening snap
	With bell, low-pitched rumbling **mid-diastolic murmur** at apex
	? Murmur of tricuspid regurgitation
Lung bases	Usually clear
Ankle oedema	Yes, if right heart failure present

Teaching Points

Causes Essentially only one – Rheumatic Fever
N.B. Rheumatic mitral stenosis is much commoner in women

Comment

If asked for details of treatment mention digoxin for associated atrial fibrillation, anticoagulants to prevent systemic embolisation from left atrial thrombus and diuretics for any associated right heart failure, as well as mitral valvotomy and mitral valve replacement.

CASE 22: MITRAL REGURGITATION

Introduce and expose
Observe

Hands	Splinters
Pulse	Sinus rhythm or Atrial fibrillation
BP	
Neck	
Face	
Praecordium	
Inspect	Visible apex beat
Palpate	Displaced / **Thrusting** apex beat / Systolic thrill Parasternal heave (due to large left atrium)
Auscultate	Soft 1st heart sound / **3rd heart sound** / **pansystolic murmur** at apex / Radiation to **axilla**
Lung bases	
Ankle oedema	

Teaching Points

Causes

1. **Ischaemic heart disease**	Secondary to left ventricular dilatation (functional) Papillary muscle ischaemia / Infarction
2. **Rheumatic heart disease**	(Previous mitral valvotomy for mitral stenosis)
3. Mitral valve prolapse	
4. Infective endocarditis	

There are many others: e.g. the connective tissue diseases (SLE, RA), Ankylosing spondylitis, Marfan's, HOCM and more.

Comment

It is sometimes difficult to give a definitive diagnosis when listening to an ejection systolic / pansystolic murmur so be sure to work out the features of the four main differential murmurs, AS / MR / Aortic sclerosis / VSD.

CASE 23: AORTIC STENOSIS

Introduce and expose	
Observe	Male
Hands	
Pulse	Sinus rhythm
BP	Low systolic with **Narrow Pulse Pressure** e.g. 110/90
Neck	Carotid pulse **Low-volume / Slow-rising** / Thrill
Face	
Praecordium	
Inspect	Visible apex beat
Palpate	Undisplaced **heaving** apex beat **Thrill** over aortic area
Auscultate	Harsh **Ejection Systolic Murmur** loudest in aortic area Often heard easily at apex / Radiates to **Carotids** Soft second heart sound (may be absent)
Lung bases	Normal if uncomplicated case
Pedal oedema	

Teaching Points

Symptoms

1. Chest pain
2. Shortness of breath
3. Syncope

Causes

1. Bicuspid valve and degeneration
2. Rheumatic
3. Congenital (young patient)

Investigations

ECG (Left ventricular hypertrophy) / CXR
Echocardiogram
Cardiac catheterisation

Comment

In the elderly, calcification of a normal valve can produce a murmur which is very similar, but the pulse, BP and apex will be normal – so called ***aortic sclerosis.***

Bicuspid valve occurs in 1% of the population, and is commoner in males. With increasing age the valve becomes increasingly fibrotic and calcified, and hence aortic stenosis most commonly presents in men aged 40–60 years.

CASE 24: AORTIC REGURGITATION

Introduce and expose	
Observe	Check for features of Marfan's* / Ankylosing spondylitis
Hands	Splinters / Rheumatoid hands / Arachnodactyly
Pulse	Sinus rhythm / **COLLAPSING**
BP	**Wide pulse pressure**, e.g. 180/60
Neck	Large volume carotid pulse / Easily seen in neck (Not JVP)
Face	High-arched palate / Argyll-Robertson pupils **(63)**
Praecordium	
Inspect	Visible apex beat
Palpate	Displaced / **Thrusting** apex beat
Auscultate	Soft / Blowing **Early Diastolic Murmur** at the left sternal edge Loudest sitting forward in held expiration **N.B.** There is always, in addition, a systolic murmur due to the increased flow across the aortic valve. There may be a mid to late diastolic murmur (Austin Flint) due to the back flow onto the mitral valve.
Lung bases	Normal in the uncomplicated case
Ankle oedema	

*High arched palate / Span > Height / Arachnodactyly / Risk of aortic dissection

Teaching Points

Causes
1. Rheumatic Fever
2. Infective Endocarditis
3. Ankylosing Spondylitis
4. Rheumatoid Arthritis
5. Marfan's Syndrome
6. Syphilis

Comment

There are a number of eponymous signs characteristic of, though rarely seen in aortic regurgitation. They are beloved by examiners!

De Musset's sign: the head nods with each pulsation.

Quincke's sign: capillary pulsation visible in the nailbeds.

Corrigan's sign: vigorous arterial pulsations seen in the neck.

CASE 25: MIXED MITRAL VALVE DISEASE

It is quite common, at least in exams, to see patients with mixed mitral valve disease, i.e. with signs of both mitral stenosis and mitral regurgitation.
Remember that, as for lone mitral stenosis, rheumatic heart disease is essentially the only cause.

Two reasons for mixed mitral valve disease:
1. Excessive valvular damage
2. Previous mitral valvotomy – **look for the lateral thoracotomy scar**

If you are doing particularly well (or you are particularly unlucky!), you may be asked to comment on the predominant valve lesion.

	Predominant MS	***Predominant MR***
Apex	Tapping	Displaced / Thrusting
1st Heart Sound	Loud	Soft
3rd Heart Sound	Absent	Present
Atrial fibrillation	Common	

Comment

Remember: 3rd heart sound represents rapid ventricular filling, and therefore is obviously incompatible with significant mitral stenosis.

CASE 26: MIXED AORTIC VALVE DISEASE

Essentially two causes:
1. Rheumatic heart disease
2. Infective endocarditis on a previously stenotic valve

Remember: even in lone aortic regurgitation you should expect to hear a systolic murmur due to increased flow across the valve. However, there will not be any signs of aortic stenosis.

		Predominant AS	*Predominant AR*
Pulse		Slow-rising	Collapsing
Apex		Heaving	Displaced / Thrusting
BP	**Systolic Pressure**	Low	High
	Pulse Pressure	Narrow	Wide

Comment

A bisferiens pulse is characteristic of mixed aortic valve disease.

CASE 27: ATRIAL FIBRILLATION

As a short 'short' case, this can occur on its own, but beware of mitral stenosis and hyperthyroidism.
If AF alone, you are likely to be asked to just feel the pulse (± apex), and you may well be asked for causes.

Introduce and expose

Observe	? obviously hyperthyroid
Hands	Sweating / Tremor
Pulse	**Irregularly irregular** in rhythm and in volume (? rate over one full minute)
BP	
Neck	Goitre
Face	Malar flush
Praecordium	
Inspect	
Palpate	
Auscultate	Again count rate over a full minute Note varying intensity of 1st heart sound
Lung bases	
Ankle oedema	

Teaching Points

Causes
1. Ischaemic heart disease
2. Mitral valve disease
3. Hyperthyroidism
4. Pneumonia
5. Cardiomyopathy
6. Constrictive pericarditis
7. 'Lone'

+ many others

Comment

*The presence of a Pulse – Apex deficit means that the atrial fibrillation is **uncontrolled**.*
***Digoxin** – the usual treatment does not alter the underlying rhythm, but simply controls the ventricular rate.*
Patients with non-rheumatic AF should be anticoagulated to decrease the risk of future stroke.

CASE 28: VENTRICULAR SEPTAL DEFECT

This is the commonest congenital heart lesion; the patient is often young.

Introduce and expose	
Observe	Young, generally well
Hands	Splinters (Rare)
Pulse	
BP	
Neck	
Face	
Praecordium	
Inspect	
Palpate	Apex undisplaced / Systolic thrill at left sternal edge
Auscultation	Loud **'tearing' pansystolic murmur** at left sternal edge / Heard well at apex
Lung bases	
Ankle oedema	

Teaching Points

1. Small VSDs (**Maladie de Roger**) in the absence of symptoms and complications, require no treatment.

2. With larger VSDs expect the apex to be displaced, with signs of **pulmonary hypertension** (RV heave / Loud P2 / Occasionally the EDM of pulmonary regurgitation). These cases will require cardiac catheterisation and surgical treatment.

3. A very large VSD can lead to **Eisenmenger's syndrome** (severe pulmonary hypertension with reversal of the shunt to R > L most often in a young patient). The massively increased blood flow irreversibly damages the pulmonary vessels. The patient will be cyanosed and display finger clubbing. The signs will be those of severe pulmonary hypertension, and the PSM tends to disappear as the right and left ventricular pressures equalise.

CASE 29: PROSTHETIC HEART VALVES

Prosthetic valves produce a loud closing click and a quieter opening click. A flow murmur across a prosthetic valve is to be expected.

Introduce and expose

Observe	Dyspnoea
Hands	Splinter haemorrhages
Pulse	Atrial fibrillation (Mitral valve replacement) Collapsing pulse – Aortic valve leaking
BP	Wide pulse pressure – Aortic valve leaking
Face	
Neck	
Praecordium	
Inspect	Midline thoracotomy scar (both aortic and mitral)
Palpate	
Auscultate	Mitral valve: loud click at 1st heart sound, opening click in diastole +/- mid-diastolic flow murmur. A Pansystolic murmur and signs of heart failure imply valve leakage. Aortic valve: normal 1st heart sound, ejection click, an ejection systolic flow murmur and loud click at 2nd heart sound. A collapsing pulse, wide pulse pressure and early diastolic murmur imply valve leakage.
Lung bases	
Ankle oedema	

Teaching Points

Complications

- Endocarditis
- Emboli
- Leakage / CCF
- Mechanical dysfunction
- Haemolysis
- Bleeding due to anticoagulants

Comment

Confusion may be caused if both valves have been replaced. An aortic valve may have been replaced by a pig graft; this does not give rise to abnormal sounds. Always comment on whether the valve is functioning normally (a flow murmur is allowed) or whether it is complicated by Leakage / CCF / Endocarditis.

CASE 30: CONGESTIVE CARDIAC FAILURE

Cardiac failure can be divided into **Left Heart Failure** where the predominant features are due to poor cardiac output and back pressure on the lungs and **Right Heart Failure** where the features are due to back pressure on the peripheral venous system. The combination of these, i.e. **Biventricular Failure**, is termed **Congestive Cardiac Failure**.

Introduce and expose

Observe	**Dyspnoea** / Oedema
Hands	Cool / Peripheral cyanosis
Pulse	Tachycardia / Poor volume
BP	Low
Neck	JVP raised **(56)**, may be behind ear
Face	
Praecordium	
Palpate	Displaced apex beat
Auscultate	3rd +/ 4th heart sounds 'Functional murmurs' of mitral and/or tricuspid regurgitation
Lung bases	Inspiratory crackles / Pleural effusion Sacral oedema
Ankle oedema	Yes – may extend as far as trunk / chest wall

Teaching Points

Causes	Ischaemic Heart Disease Valvular heart disease Cardiomyopathy (Dilated / Restrictive / HOCM) Arrhythmias

---

Comment

High output cardiac failure refers to conditions in which the heart fatigues after excessive pumping of blood, as in arteriovenous shunts or anaemia. It is very uncommon and is almost best forgotten.

RESPIRATORY SYSTEM

"Examine this Patient's Chest"

When asked to examine the chest there are only a few possible diagnoses and you should be able to differentiate between them fairly easily. However, many candidates look ill-prepared when it comes to the exam. It is very important to have a strict, well-practised routine (as in all short cases). Examination is in six main parts:

Introduce and expose

	Remove shirt / blouse (preserve modesty) and sit up at 45 degrees	
Observe	Dyspnoea / Respiratory rate Ask the patient to take two deep breaths Watch from halfway down the bed for: 1. Asymmetry of chest movement 2. Stridor 3. Cachexia 4. Accessory muscle use / Pursed lips	
Hands	Clubbing	Tumour / Pus (Bronchiectasis, abscess) / Fibrosing alveolitis
	Asterixis	Hypercapnia
	Tremor	Beta-Agonist esp. Nebulised
	Tar Staining	Smoker
	Steroidal skin	Steroid use in chronic bronchitis / Fibrosing alveolitis / asthma
	Pulse	Hyperdynamic / Tachycardia
	HPOA **(3)**	Tender on squeezing wrist (Usually clubbed)
Face	Central cyanosis	Look at tongue
	Cushingoid **(92)**	
	Horner's syndrome **(61)**	Apical lung tumour
Neck	Trachea	Pulled to side of collapse / Pushed away from mass / fluid
	JVP	Raised and pulsatile – Cor pulmonale Raised and fixed – SVCO **(33)**
	Lymphadenopathy See also cases **(54–56)**	

Chest You have to decide whether to examine the front or the back first. We would suggest the back as usually all of the possible signs will be there; if so, you may be told to omit the front thus saving valuable time and not boring the examiner.

Expansion	Make sure your thumbs are not touching the chest
Percussion	Top to bottom including axillae
Tactile Vocal Fremitus (TVF)	Use the ulnar border of both hands
Auscultation	Start at apex
Vocal resonance (VR)	

TVF and VR give the same information. VR is more reliable. You may wish to omit TVF to save time but you should be able to justify your actions.

Ankle oedema

Extras

Oxygen	
Nebulisers / Inhalers	
Sputum pot	Purulent = Infection / Abscess / Bronchiectasis Blood = Tumour / Infection
Temperature chart	

Comment

At the end of the examination you should be in a position to make a differential diagnosis of the lung pathology. Try also to note whether there is right heart failure (Cor pulmonale). E.g. "This lady is breathless at rest and has signs of lower zone fibrosis consistent with a diagnosis of fibrosing alveolitis. There is no evidence of right heart failure" or "The raised JVP and ankle oedema suggest this has been complicated by pulmonary hypertension".

CASE 31: PLEURAL EFFUSION

This is a common short case and should be well performed.

Introduce and expose

Observe	Chest movement less on affected side / **Cachexia** / Radiotherapy marks Mastectomy / Aspiration scars (under the plaster!)
Hands	**Clubbing (43)** / Tar stains / Rheumatoid
Face	Cyanosis / SLE butterfly rash
Neck	Lymphadenopathy / Trachea (away from large effusion but towards if coexisting lung collapse)
Chest	Decreased TVF / **stony dull percussion** **Decreased BS** / Decreased VF May have bronchial breathing at upper limit of effusion
Extras	TB (Asian) / Temp chart / Sputum (blood stained) / Ankles (Oedema-CCF / DVT-PE)

Teaching Points

Causes	Exudate (protein >30g/l)	Transudate (protein <30g/l)
	Tumour (Primary / Secondary) Pulmonary embolus/infarction Pneumonia TB SLE / Rheumatoid Diaphragmatic irritation (Abscess / Pancreatitis)	Cardiac failure **(30)** Nephrotic syndrome **(11)** Cirrhosis **(6)**

Comment

There are many rarer causes. Mesothelioma is usually associated with clubbing and occurs more often after asbestos exposure.

Investigations would include: *CXR / Sputum cytology / Sputum MCS*
Pleural fluid analysis /
Pleural biopsy.

Treatment would include symptomatic drainage and treatment of the underlying condition.

CASE 32: FIBROSING ALVEOLITIS

Introduce and expose

Observe	Dyspnoea / Accessory muscle use / Tachypnoea
Hands	**Clubbing** (60%)
Face	Central Cyanosis (if advanced)
Neck	
Chest	Breath sounds – **fine inspiratory crackles** **Bases** > Apex
Extras	Oxygen / Cushingoid / Steroidal skin Ask to see FEV_1 and FVC measurements

Teaching Points

Other causes of lung fibrosis

Widespread	**Upper**	**Lower**
Drugs *Busulphan* *Amiodarone* Carcinomatosis Extrinsic Allergic Alveolitis	TB **(34)** Radiation (Ca Breast) Ankylosing spondylitis	Sarcoidosis Asbestosis Chronic pulmonary oedema Mitral valve disease **(21)** Silicosis Rheumatoid / SLE **(8,9)**

Comment

FEV_1 and FVC are both reduced causing a restrictive pulmonary deficit. In the absence of an underlying diagnosis, cryptogenic fibrosing alveolitis is the name given. However, there are many autoimmune disorders that are complicated by a similar pulmonary disorder: Rheumatoid, SLE, Systemic Sclerosis, Sjögren's, Polymyositis and Chronic Active Hepatitis. Look out for signs of these.

CASE 33: SUPERIOR VENA CAVAL OBSTRUCTION (SVCO)

Introduce and expose

Observe	Stridor / Dyspnoea
Hands	Clubbed / Tar stained
Face	**Oedematous** / Cyanosed / Puffy eyes
Neck	**Fixed engorged veins** / Lymphadenopathy
Chest	Tortuous veins / Signs of tumour
Extras	Horner's syndrome / Radiation marks

Teaching Points

Causes **Carcinoma of bronchus**
Lymphoma
Mediastinal goitre / Fibrosis

Comment

*Urgent treatment with radiotherapy or stenting is required. The patient may complain of **Headaches / Lightheadedness / Syncope**.*

CASE 34: OLD TB

Introduce and expose

Observe	Patient elderly / Asian / Irish / Abnormal shaped chest
Hands	
Face	
Neck	**Trachea to side of collapse**
Chest	Decreased expansion / Old thoracotomy scar / Rib missing TVF may be decreased PN Dull **BS Crackles** (bronchial breathing) VF Decreased

Teaching Points

The signs are very variable but are due to **fibrosis and scarring**, leaving areas without working lung tissue. The apex of the lung is most often affected but the signs of apical disease can be difficult to pick up. Beware!

Complications	Fungal mycetoma in cavities Malignant change in old scar tissue

---

Comment

Prior to anti-TB drugs pneumothorax, plombage (ping-pong balls put into the chest cavity) and phrenic nerve crush were all used in the treatment of TB. Signs of these may be visible.

ABDOMINAL SYSTEM
"Examine this Patient's Abdomen"

The key to a successful examination of the abdomen is to look for any extra-abdominal signs to indicate whether there is a problem with liver function, haematological function or both and then go on to find any abdominal signs. By the end of the examination you should be able to tie the two together.

Introduce and expose

Observe	Jaundice	Liver failure
	Wasting	Malabsorption / Malignancy
	Purpura	Hypersplenism
	Pigmentation	Haemochromatosis / Multiple transfusions
	Tattoos	Risk of hepatitis
	Polycythaemia	Polycystic kidneys
	Hyperventilating	Acidosis (Renal failure)
Hands	Clubbing	Inflammatory Bowel Disease
	Leuconychia	Low serum albumin
	Spider naevi	Liver dysfunction
	Asterixis / Tremor	"
	Palmar erythema	"
	Dupuytren's	Alcohol / Phenytoin etc.
	Bruising	Clotting function impaired
	Arteriovenous fistula for dialysis (forearm)	
Face	Cushingoid (Steroids)	Chronic Active Hepatitis Transplant Inflammatory Bowel Disease
	Kayser-Fleischer rings	Wilson's disease
	Jaundice	
	Xanthelasma	Primary Biliary Cirrhosis Chronic Biliary Obstruction
	Steroidal	
	Mouth ulcers	
	Parotid enlargement	Alcoholism
Neck	Lymphadenopathy	(Virchow's node)
	Neck feeding line	Malabsorption
	Dialysis line	Polycystic kidneys

Chest	Spider naevi	
	Gynaecomastia	(decreased breakdown of oestrogens)
	Sit forward and look for Scars / Sacral oedema / More spider naevi	

Now ask the patient to lie as flat as possible / comfortable, one pillow. Get down to the patient's level.

Abdomen	Do not hurt the patient
	Ask permission / Ask if tender
Inspect	Masses / Ascites / Scars / Striae / Visible peristalsis
	Dilated veins
Palpate	Ask if there is any tenderness before touching
	Masses Liver / Spleen / Kidneys (see below)
	Inguinal nodes / Herniae
Percuss	Delineate size of masses
	Shifting dullness (Ascites) / No need to turn patient if not dull
Auscultate	Bowel sounds
	Are there any bruits over Liver / Mass / Renal artery / Aortic aneurysm

Tell the examiner that "to complete my examination I would usually examine the external genitalia and perform a rectal examination".

Legs	Ankle oedema	Low protein states
	Bruising	
	Erythema nodosum	Crohn's / Ulcerative Colitis (7)
	Neuropathy	Alcohol / B12 deficiency (Do not routinely examine for this but if there is muscle wasting suggest that you would)

Extras	Asterixis	Encephalopathy
	Urine	Bile / Protein / Blood
	Temperature chart	Infection
	Scratch marks	Cholestasis

CASE 35: HEPATOMEGALY

Introduce and expose

Inspect — Distension in Right Hypochondrium

Striae	Chronic liver disease / Obesity
Scars	Previous tumours (? liver metastases) Transplant / Shunts
Ascites	
Stoma	Ulcerative colitis and sclerosing cholangitis / Tumours (mets)

Palpate — Start at Right Iliac Fossa and move up
Describe liver edge

Smooth	Normal / Hepatitis / CCF
Nodular	Mets / Cirrhosis / Tumour
Pulsatile	Tricuspid regurgitation
Tender	Cardiac failure / Hepatitis

Percuss — Upper and lower borders, measure size in mid clavicular line. Normal=12cm

Auscultate — Bruit Hepatocellular carcinoma (in chronic cirrhosis). Often mistermed hepatoma. N.B. it is not benign.
Tricuspid regurgitation
Arteriovenous malformation

Don't forget the rest of the abdomen.

Teaching Points

Causes

The **3 Cs**
- **Carcinomatosis** / Hepatocellular carcinoma
- **Congestive Cardiac Failure** (JVP, ankle oedema) **(30)**
- **Cirrhosis**

Others
- Fatty infiltration (alcohol)
- Myeloproliferative disease
- Haemochromatosis (pigmented, diabetic)
- Lymphoproliferative disease
- Infection (hepatitis, glandular fever, HIV, hydatid)
- Biliary obstruction
- Infiltrates (sarcoid, amyloid)

Comment

At the end of the examination you should be able to tell the examiner that "there is isolated hepatomegaly with (or without) decompensation of liver function". You should comment on any features that will lead you to a more definitive diagnosis.

CASE 36: SPLENOMEGALY

Inspect	Swelling / Bruising / Purpura
Palpate	Start in Right iliac fossa and move across
	Note edge and notch
	Mass moves down with respiration
	Unable to palpate above (not ballottable)
Percuss	Dull (no bowel gas above)
	Dullness up to 9th rib / Mid axillary line
Auscultate	Feel for any other lymph nodes / Cervical / Axillary / Inguinal / Epitrochlear etc.

Teaching Points

Causes

Myeloproliferative disease	**Chronic Myeloid Leukaemia**
	Myelofibrosis
Lymphoproliferative disease	**Chronic Lymphatic Leukaemia**
	Lymphoma
	Myelomatosis
	Acute Lymphatic Leukaemia
Portal hypertension	**Cirrhosis**
	Hepatic vein obstruction
Infection	**Glandular fever** / Bacterial endocarditis
Infiltrates	Sarcoid / Amyloid

Comment

There are many more causes of spleen and liver enlargement. You should know and suggest the more common ones as possible diagnoses.

CASE 37: HEPATOSPLENOMEGALY

You must go over all the points covered during isolated liver or spleen enlargement. It may be difficult to distinguish between massive hepatomegaly and hepatosplenomegaly. Check to see if the splenic dullness behind the ribs continues over the abdomen, if not it is more likely to be hepatomegaly alone.

Teaching Points

Causes Myeloproliferative disease
Lymphoproliferative disease (? other lymph nodes)
Cirrhosis with portal hypertension
Beta-thalassaemia (iron deposition in skin, young)

CASE 38: ASCITES

This may appear as part of chronic liver disease or in isolation, in which case you must know the most common causes.

Inspect	Swelling / Vein distension / Everted umbilicus
Palpate	Tense / Organs may be hard to feel
	Fluctuation
	Fluid thrill
Percuss	Stony dull in flanks / Shifting dullness

Teaching Points

Causes **Cirrhosis** with portal hypertension / Chronic liver disease **(6)**
Malignancy GI / Liver mets / Ovary
Right sided heart failure
Nephrotic syndrome **(11)**
Many others!

CASE 39: RENAL MASSES

There are three main possibilities:

Unilateral enlargement
Bilateral enlargement
Transplanted kidney

The extra abdominal signs should be noted prior to examining the abdomen.

Inspect	Scars in loin / Transplant in groin Scars from previous CAPD catheters Arteriovenous fistula in arm
Palpate	Bimanual palpation of mass in loin (ballottable) Able to get above it A transplanted kidney is found in the iliac fossa, dull to percussion (be careful with it!)
Percuss	Resonant (due to bowel gas between kidney and skin)
Ausculte	Bruit Tumour / Renal artery stenosis

Teaching Points

Causes	Polycystic kidneys (only one may be palpable) Malignancy Hydronephrosis Hypertrophy of single or single functioning kidney Renal cyst

---

Comment

Polycystic kidneys show autosomal dominant inheritance. Cysts are also found in many other organs, especially the liver, spleen and pancreas. Subarachnoid haemorrhage occurs in 5–10% of patients.

"Examine this Patient's Hands"

There are many diagnoses that may be picked up when you are asked to look at a patient's hands. You must develop a thorough routine so as not to miss any important signs.

Introduce and expose

Observe	**General**		Cachexia
			Psoriatic skin rash
	Face	Cushingoid	Rheumatoid / SLE (may have Carpal Tunnel Syndrome)
		Exophthalmos	Thyroid acropachy **(14)**
		Acromegaly	CTS / Diabetic neuropathy / Thickened nerves
		Heliotrope	Dermatomyositis **(47)**
Hands	**Nails**	Clubbing **(43)**	
		Splinter haemorrhages	Endocarditis **(2)**
		Leuconychia	Low protein states
		Nail bed infarcts	Rheumatoid **(8,40)** / Systemic sclerosis
		Pitting, ridging etc.	Psoriasis
	Skin	Tight	Scleroderma / CREST **(45)**
		Steroidal	
		Raynaud's phenomenon	
		Spider naevi	
		Gouty tophi	
		Rash of dermatomyositis	
		Palmar pigmentation **(95)**	
		Tendon xanthomata	
	Joints	Observe	Swelling / Deformity / Inflammation
		Palpate	Tenderness / Synovial thickening
			Heberden's / Osler's nodes
	Nerves	Wasting	Interossei / Thenar / Hypothenar
		Weakness	1st dorsal interosseous – Ulnar
			Abductor pollicis brevis – Median
		Sensation	Pin Prick / JPS / Vib
			Differentiate between Ulnar / Median / Radial / C6 C7 C8
	Function	Undo and do up button / Write / Hold cup etc.	

Palms Rheumatoid nodules / Dupuytren's contracture / Erythema

Wrists Peripheral pulses

Elbows Gouty tophi / Rheumatoid nodules
Psoriatic plaques
Tendon xanthomata

CASE 40: RHEUMATOID HANDS

Introduce and expose

Observe Wasting / Cushingoid

Hands **Ask if hands are painful**

Nails — Nail bed infarcts

Skin — Steroidal / Raynaud's / Ulcers over nodules

Joints — Symmetrical disease
Soft tissue swelling / Spindling of fingers
Swelling / Redness / Synovitis / especially Metacarpo-phalangeal joints
Ulnar deviation of fingers
Swan neck deformity
Boutonnière deformity
Z deformity of thumb
Subluxation of proximal phalanx

Nerves Wasting of small muscles of hand / Generalised weakness
No movement if tendon ruptured
Grip strength decreased with severity
Change if coexisting CTS / Polyneuropathy / Ulnar entrapment at elbow

Function May be markedly decreased

Extras **Nodules** over tendons particularly at elbows

See also **(8)**.

CASE 41: OSTEOARTHRITIS

Introduce and expose
Observe

Hands	**Nails**	
	Skin	
	Joints	Heberden's nodes (Bony swelling of Distal IPJs) Bouchard's nodes (Bony swelling of Proximal IPJs) Squaring of hands (1st Carpometacarpal joint)
Nerves		
Function		May be decreased

<u>**Teaching Points**</u>

Primary	Middle aged women / Familial / esp. DIPJ involvement	
Secondary	Many causes of joint damage	
	Wear and Tear / Trauma	Heavy lifting / Runners etc.
	Disabled patients	In arm of crutch use
	Inflammatory arthritides	RA (**40**) / Gout (**46**) / Others
	Neuropathic (Charcot) joints	

CASE 42: PSORIASIS

You may come across this either when asked to examine the hands or to comment on the rash. Invariably, one will lead on to the other.

Introduce and expose

Observe		Generalised skin changes
Hands	**Nails**	Pitting / Ridging / Onycholysis / Hyperkeratosis / Discolouration
	Skin	Plaques
		Sausage shaped fingers
	Joints	Distal interphalangeal joint swelling
		Rheumatoid pattern (symmetrical small joint swelling)
		Arthritis mutilans (telescoping of phalanges)
		Monarthritis of larger joints
		Ankylosing spondylitis / Sacroiliitis type
	Rash	Salmon pink plaques / Silver white scales
		Look or ask to see Extensor surfaces / Scalp / Navel / Natal cleft

Comment

There are several types of skin lesion: Chronic plaques, Guttate, Pustular and Erythrodermic. Many drugs can exacerbate the condition including: Alcohol / Beta-Blockers / NSAIDs / Lithium.

CASE 43: CLUBBING

Introduce and expose

Observe	Signs of underlying disease
Hands	**Loss of angle** at the nail bed
	Increased curvature of the nail
	Fluctuation of the nail bed

When discussing the possible underlying causes you must look for any pointers that may give you the diagnosis in that patient.

Teaching Points

Causes

Lung	Carcinoma of the bronchus	Tar stains / Cachexia
	Fibrosing alveolitis	Dyspnoea
	Bronchiectasis	Sputum pot
	Mesothelioma	
Bowel	Cirrhosis	Signs of liver disease
	Inflammatory bowel disease	Wasted
Heart	Endocarditis	Splinter haemorrhages
	Cyanotic congenital heart disease	Down's syndrome
	Myxoma	
Thyroid	Acropachy	Exophthalmos / Goitre
Hereditary	Idiopathic	

CASE 44: ULNAR / MEDIAN / TI LESIONS

	ULNAR	MEDIAN	T1
Observe	Clawing 4th and 5th fingers		
Wasted muscles	Hypothenar Interossei	Thenar	All small muscles
Weakness	Add / Abduction of fingers	Abductor pollicis brevis	All
Sensory Loss	Medial 1.5 digits	Lateral 3.5 digits	Medial forearm
Extras	Deformed elbow Rheumatoid	Tinel's sign at wrist over Carpal tunnel Scar at wrist	Neck Lymphadenopathy Ipsilateral Horner's

Teaching Points

Causes

The median and ulnar nerves may be damaged anywhere along their course due to trauma. Common sites of entrapment are: the carpal tunnel (Median), the elbow in patients with rheumatoid arthritis (Median and/or Ulnar). The nerves can of course be individually affected by a mononeuropathy.

T1 root lesions may be due to damage anywhere along its course:

Cord (Esp. bilateral)	Syringomyelia (**84**) / Tumour
Root	Cervical spondylosis
Plexus	Pancoast tumour (assn. Horner's syndrome (**61**)) / Cachexia etc)

Comment

*A radial nerve lesion is less common. The clinical features are sensory loss over the lateral dorsum of the hand and adjacent forearm, and motor weakness involving the extensors of the wrist and fingers, supinator and the extensor carpi radialis, giving **Wrist Drop.***

CASE 45: SCLERODERMA / CREST

Although rare in clinical practice this is commonly seen in examinations.

Introduce and expose		
Observe	**General**	(Signs of Mixed Connective Tissue Disease **(9)**)
	Face	Tight skin around mouth / Telangiectasia / Dry eyes
Hands	**Skin**	Tight / Shiny / Spindle shaped fingers / Calcinosis / Raynaud's / Pulp infarcts / Autoamputation
	Nails	Nail bed infarcts
	Joints	Swollen
	Nerves	Usually none / Carpal tunnel / Proximal muscle weakness **(87)**
	Function	May be severely restricted
Arms	Skin changes may occur over much of the body surface.	

Teaching Points

Systemic sclerosis is a multisystem disease and although the skin changes are the most obvious manifestation, joint, gastrointestinal, renal and cardiorespiratory complications are the main causes of morbidity and mortality.

Comment

One of the most troublesome features is coldness. The patient may have battery heated gloves.

CASE 46: GOUT

TOPHACEOUS GOUT

Introduce and expose		
Observe	Obesity / Ruddy 'Boozers' face	
Hands	Nails	
	Skin	Thin or ulcerated over tophi (subcutaneous yellow/white nodules)
	Joints	**Asymmetrical** swelling of small joints Tophi over joints
	Nerves	Associated carpal tunnel syndrome **(44)**
Elbows	Tophi	
Function	May be decreased depending on severity	
Extras	Look for tophi on ear Similar picture on the feet	

Teaching Points

Differential diagnosis at elbow	Rheumatoid nodules
Complications	Renal stones Carpal tunnel syndrome

Comment

Occasionally there is gross deformity of the joints due to tophus formation and joint margin erosions. Uric acid crystals are needle shaped and negatively birefringent. Treatment of the acute attack is with NSAIDs and of the chronic condition with allopurinol.

GOUT – SINGLE JOINT

You may be asked to comment on a single inflamed joint (Red / Tender / Swollen).
The hallux is the joint most often affected.

Teaching Points

Precipitating factors	Drugs: aspirin / diuretics / allopurinol Stress / Surgery Exercise

CASE 47: DERMATOMYOSITIS

Introduce and expose

Observe	Cachexia	
Face	Heliotrope rash around eyes with mild oedema	
Hands	Nails	Rash around nail bed
	Skin	Purple rash over knuckles (extensor surface of elbows and knees)
	Raynaud's phenomenon	
Other	Proximal muscle weakness and muscle tenderness	

Teaching Points

M:F 2:1
Malignancy 30% age 30, 40% age 40, 50% age 50 etc.
Overlap with Mixed Connective Tissue Disease **(9)**

Investigation Serum creatine kinase and ESR increased
EMG changes
Muscle biopsy

Treatment Oral steroids

Comments

Polymyositis is a similar condition which includes the muscle weakness and tenderness without the skin changes (87).

SKIN
"Look at this Patient's Rash"

Skin diseases often cause confusion amongst students, mainly due to the extra terms that dermatologists use to describe lesions. To 'demystify' dermatology we think it is useful to describe a skin lesion as any surgical lump (this is something that should be second nature by the time of finals) and then use specific terms when needed. The features of a lump that should be described are given below, some specific dermatological terms are also given. It is not necessary to use these all the time but when used appropriately it shows a greater understanding on your part.

Colour	Erythema	Increased perfusion
Shape	Plaque	Flat topped disc
	Macule	Flat area of discolouration
Size	Papule	<1 cm of elevated skin
	Nodule	>1 cm palpable mass
Surface	Vesicle	Blister <5 mm
	Bulla	Blister >5 mm
	Pustule	Blister containing pus
	Scale	Flaky keratin
	Crust	Dried exudate
Site	Exact position if localised	
	? Flexor or Extensor if generalised	
Edge		

In the case of an **ulcer** you should describe the **Edge / Base / Depth / Discharge / Surrounding tissues.**

To practice describing skin lesions, look at a colour atlas of dermatology and go through how you would present a similar case if you saw it in the exam.

There are only a finite number of skin lesions and those likely to come up as a short case are even fewer. Systemic diseases that have cutaneous manifestations or dermatological conditions that have systemic complications are the most common short cases and you should be aware of these. Primary dermatological diseases are unlikely to come up unless a patient happens to have coexisting eczema.

You should be familiar with the following rashes / skin lesions and their systemic diseases:

Skin Sign	Disease
Dermatitis herpetiformis	Coeliac disease
Lupus pernio / Nodules	Sarcoidosis
Necrobiosis lipoidica **(50)**	Diabetes
Pretibial myxoedema **(49)**	Graves' disease
Erythema nodosum **(48)**	Many
Hereditary haemorrhagic telangiectasiae **(96)**	Blood loss (GI / Lung)
Acanthosis nigricans	Malignancy / Diabetes / Cushing's
Vitiligo **(53)**	Many
Lupus	Discoid / Systemic **(9)**
Neurofibromatosis **(100)**	Many systemic complications
Adenoma sebaceum etc.	Tuberose sclerosis (Epilepsy / Low IQ)
Port wine stain	Sturge-Weber (Epilepsy)
Erythema multiforme **(52)**	Infections / Drugs
Purpura	Haematological problems
Erythema ab igne **(51)**	Pain ? Cause

Tendon xanthomata / Xanthelasma / Eruptive xanthomata / Palmar xanthomata are associated with different hyperlipidaemias. Be sure to know which skin lesion is which.

Other common skin problems include

Ulcers	Venous	
	Ischaemic	Rheumatoid / Sickle / Vascular insufficiency
	Neuropathic	
Eczema		
Psoriasis		**(42)**
Lichen planus		Itchy wrists / Wickham's striae in mouth
Pityriasis rosea		Oval lesions on trunk / Herald patch
Pityriasis versicolor		**(53)**
Rosacea		Facial papules / Pustules / Telangiectasia Eye Blepharitis / Conjunctivitis / Iritis
Shingles		Herpes zoster (common) Erythematous rash over dermatome / Associated pain

CASE 48: ERYTHEMA NODOSUM

Site	Shins (occasionally thighs)
Description	Tender / red / raised lesions 2–6 cm in diameter
Causes	Sarcoidosis Streptococcal infection Drugs (Sulphonamides / Penicillin / Oral Contraceptive) Inflammatory Bowel Disease Primary TB Pregnancy Rheumatic fever Many others

CASE 49: PRETIBIAL MYXOEDEMA

Site	Shins (+/- feet)
Description	Raised / purple-red lesions with 'orange peel' appearance If severe, skin thickened with non-pitting oedema
Cause	**Graves' Disease (14)**

Note: Pretibial myxoedema usually develops after the hyperthyroidism has been treated.
Look for exophthalmos or a thyroidectomy scar.

CASE 50: NECROBIOSIS LIPOIDICA

Site Shins (occasionally arms)

Description Shiny yellow plaques with waxy centre
Brown-red margins and nearby telangiectasiae

Cause **Diabetes mellitus (13)**
Look for tell-tale signs on patient's bedside locker – BM stix / sugar-free juice / diabetic chocolate etc.

CASE 51: ERYTHEMA AB IGNE

Site Commonly shins, or lateral aspect of one leg, from sitting next to the fire. Also low back, from exposure to hot water bottle.

Description Pigmented / Erythematous reticular discolouration

Causes Exposure to excessive heat, therefore:
- Chronic pain / Myeloma **(12)**
- Intolerance of cold (?hypothyroid)

CASE 52: ERYTHEMA MULTIFORME

Site	Limbs and trunk	
	Classically, backs of hands, forearms, feet and toes	
Description	Red papules with central pallor – 'target lesions'	
	Bullae can develop within the lesions	
Causes	Unknown (50%)	
	Infection	Herpes simplex / Mycoplasma Pneumonia
	Drugs	Sulphonamides / Penicillin
	Connective tissue diseases	
	Neoplasia	

Comment

Stevens-Johnson syndrome is a severe form, with widespread bullous eruptions and orogenital ulceration. It is potentially life-threatening.

CASE 53: VITILIGO

Site	Anywhere Often hands, face and neck, dorsum of feet
Description	Symmetrical patches of depigmentation with hyperpigmented borders
Causes	Vitiligo is associated with organ specific autoimmune diseases of which more than one may be present in an individual. Look for alopecia and ask for a family history of vitiligo or associated diseases.

Thyroid Disease	
Pernicious Anaemia	
Addison's Disease	**(95)**
Diabetes Mellitus	**(13)**
Alopecia Areata	
Chronic Active Hepatitis	
Primary Biliary Cirrhosis	
Fibrosing Alveolitis	**(32)**

PITYRIASIS VERSICOLOR

This is a skin infection caused by the yeast *Pityrosporum orbiculare (Malassezia furfur)* which may look like vitiligo. It is noticed especially when the patient has been sunbathing, with white patches on the tanned skin, but pale brown patches on the non-exposed areas.

"Examine this Patient's Neck"

This command indicates one of three possibilities:

Abnormal JVP
Cervical Lymphadenopathy
Goitre ± Abnormal thyroid status

If the patient is sitting on a chair that you can get behind and/or there is a glass of water nearby, it is most likely to be a goitre and less likely to be an abnormal JVP. If the patient is on a bed and is able to lean back the opposite is true. This is a difficult case. However, if you are methodical you will not miss anything.

Introduce and expose

Observe	**General**	Thyroid eyes – Exophthalmos / Lid retraction
		Glass of water nearby – Goitre
		Dyspnoea – Cor pulmonale (Right heart failure)
		Wasting – Malignancy / Lymphadenopathy
Inspect	**Neck**	Obvious goitre? Yes – Go on to Case **54**
		No – Go on to Case **55**

CASE 54: GOITRE

Palpate the mass as for any lump ?Single nodule / Multinodular / Diffusely enlarged
Ask the patient to swallow (having taken a sip of water and held it in their mouth).
A goitre should move up.
Palpate for any associated lymphadenopathy.

Percuss over the top of the manubrium / Dullness may indicate a retrosternal thyroid.

Auscultate over the thyroid for a bruit.

Ask the examiner if you could test the thyroid status **(14/93).**
Also ask to look for eye signs **(68)**.

Comment

*To revise the thyroid fully you must look at the four cases **14 / 54 / 68 / 93**.*

CASE 55: LYMPHADENOPATHY

Inspect	**Neck**	Obvious raised JVP?	Yes – Go to Case **56**
			No – Carry on

Ask patient to sit forward

Palpate each of the neck areas in turn **(From Behind)**.
Describe the lump or lumps as you would any 'surgical lump': Site / Shape / Surface etc.
The most common diagnoses are:

1. Reactive (Infection)
2. Neoplastic metastases
3. Lymphoma
4. Tuberculosis

If no goitre and no lymphadenopathy look carefully for the JVP.

CASE 56: JVP

It is almost impossible to describe in print the difficult job of assessing the JVP. We strongly advise you to arrange bedside teaching before the exam, which is by far the best way to understand what is going on.

Lean the patient back at 45 degrees
Look for raised JVP (may be above ear)
Measure height above the sternal angle
If not seen gently press abdomen (Ask patient)
Time pulsation against opposite carotid pulse

Big systolic V wave	CCF / Tricuspid regurgitation
Big diastolic A wave	Pulmonary hypertension
	Pulmonary / Tricuspid stenosis
	Heart Block (Unlikely in exams)

Non-Pulsatile SVCO (**33**) / Excessively high CCF (**30**)

NERVOUS SYSTEM
"Examine this Patient's Cranial Nerves"

It is not usual practice to expect a candidate to examine all twelve nerves and to look at the fundi on one request. Rather, you will be asked to look at an already dilated fundus, look at the eyes (meaning II, III, IV and VI) or examine the lower cranial nerves (meaning V–XII but not VI).
However, be prepared to start at the top and work down. You must practise cranial nerve examination many times.

I Ask the patient "Have you noticed any problems with your sense of taste or your ability to smell things?" If the answer is yes tell the examiner you would usually go on to test these sensations formally and check to see if the patient can breathe through each nostril.

Eyes Observe

Ptosis	III / Sympathetic / Myasthenia
Squint (69)	Congenital / Acquired
Exophthalmos	Thyroid ophthalmoplegia

II **Acuity** Remember that visual acuity is the single most important function of vision, without it a person is blind! Ask "Do you wear glasses or contact lenses?" If yes, ask them to put them on and tell the examiner "At this stage I usually test the visual acuity formally with a Snellen chart at six meters." He may then tell you the acuity; if not, test it with a pocket Snellen chart held at the appropriate distance (this looks more impressive than picking up the nearest newspaper). It is important to look very confident when testing acuity so practise it until you do.

Fields Test these against your own with a red hat pin. Do not forget to test for a central scotoma. Practise looking good at this as well, it is very easy to see whether a candidate has any idea of what he or she is doing.

Pupils Have a bright pen torch to test direct response and consensual response. Test the response to accommodation by asking the patient to look at the far side of the room and then at your finger which should be held 10 cm away from the patient's nose. Make sure you are in a position to see the pupillary response!

Fundi Leave this until the end.
Look at the discs followed by the rest of the fundus in a consistent order. (If you are told that the patient has decreased acuity whilst being handed an ophthalmoscope look at the macular area after the disc as this is where the pathology is most likely to be.)
Usually fundal examination is considered as a separate case.

III IV VI

Ask the patient to follow your pen torch and to tell you if he sees double. Hold it vertically when testing the medial and lateral recti and horizontally when testing the other muscles.
Comment on which muscles are not working. If it is not obvious when the patient complains of diplopia, cover up one eye and ask which image disappears (the outermost image is from the affected eye i.e. the one that has not moved).
If nystagmus is present describe which eye is affected the most and which direction the fast phase is **(64/65)**.

V

Motor Ask the patient to open his mouth (pterygoids)
Ask the patient to clench his teeth together (masseters / temporalis)

Sensory Check sensitivity to pin and touch over the three divisions
Tell the examiner "*At this stage I would usually test the corneal reflex*". It is unlikely that you will be expected to do this but you should know that the afferent limb of the reflex is trigeminal and the efferent limb is through the facial nerve to the orbicularis oculi muscles.

VII

Assess the patient's facial movements by asking him to close his eyes tightly, raise his eyebrows and show his teeth.

VIII

Ask the patient if he has any problem hearing with either ear. Rub the hair near his ear between your finger and thumb. Tuning fork tests may be needed if there is decreased hearing. Otoscopy is not expected but should be offered if there is a suggestion of a conductive defect. It is important to test hearing in any patient who has a nearby cranial nerve lesion (V / VII / IX / X) as a tumour compressing more than one nerve may be the underlying problem **(78)**.

IX X Watch for palatal movement when the patient is saying "ahh". The side that does not move is the abnormal one! Do not get into discussions of uvula movement, these only confuse the matter.
Tell the examiner "At this stage I would normally test the gag reflex in order to assess sensation". You won't usually be expected to do this.

XII Look at the tongue inside the mouth for wasting and fasciculation (lower motor neurone signs) and then ask the patient to move it. A spastic tongue will not be wasted but will move slowly.

XI Ask the patient to shrug his shoulders and then to turn his head from one side to the other whilst you palpate the sternomastoid muscles.

CASE 57: HOMONYMOUS HEMIANOPIA

General	Look for signs of hemiparesis / All on the same side! E.g. **R** HH / **R** Facial palsy / **R** Sided weakness (Unable to shake hands etc.)
Acuity	Normal
Fields	Lesion posterior to the optic chiasm Optic tract — May be asymmetrical Optic radiation — Upper quadrants Temporal lobe disease Lower quadrants Parietal lobe disease Occipital cortex ? Macular sparing
Pupils	Normal
Movements	Normal
Fundi	Normal / Papilloedema if space occupying lesion
Extras	Tell the examiner that you would like to go on and look for other focal neurological signs, especially those commonly found in CVAs (Hemiparesis on appropriate side / Neglect with Left HH / Dysphasia with Right HH)

Teaching Points

Most cases are due to cerebrovascular disease. Tumours and other space occupying lesions are less common.

Comment: Investigation

Formal perimetry / CT Brain scan
Risk factors for CVA (Hypertension / AF / Diabetes / Carotid bruits)

CASE 58: BITEMPORAL HEMIANOPIA

General	May be signs of pituitary disease (see below)
Acuity	Normal unless coexisting pressure on optic nerve
Fields	**Lesion at the chiasm** damaging crossing nasal retinal fibres
	Upper quadrant bitemporal hemianopia due to pituitary tumour damaging inferior fibres first
	Lower quadrant bitemporal hemianopia due to craniopharyngioma damaging superior fibres first
Pupils	Normal
Movements	Normal
Fundi	Optic atrophy if coexisting optic nerve compression

Teaching Points

Causes Pituitary tumour — Look for abnormal pituitary function
Craniopharyngioma / Meningioma / Aneurysm

CASE 59: CENTRAL SCOTOMA

There is a large overlap between this and optic atrophy **(72)**.

Acuity	Decreased	
Fields	**Loss of centre of visual field** with preservation of peripheral fields	
Pupils	Normal / May have afferent pupillary defect	
Movements	Normal	
Fundi	Depends on cause	Optic atrophy Macular retinal damage

Teaching Points

Causes

Primary Damage to nerve

Demyelination (20)
Compression (Tumour / Paget's disease **(101)** / Thyroid eye disease)
Ischaemic / Toxic (Methyl alcohol / Lead / Quinine)
Infective (Syphilis) / Nutritional (B12 deficiency **(88)**)
Hereditary (Friedreich's ataxia **(88)** / Leber's optic atrophy)
Glaucoma

Secondary To chronic papilloedema **(73)**

Consecutive To retinal disease: Retinitis pigmentosa; Choroiditis

CASE 60: TUNNEL VISION / CONCENTRIC CONSTRICTION

Acuity	Normal (Decreased if advanced disease)
Fields	Loss of peripheral fields with normal central field
Pupils	Normal
Movements	Normal
Fundi	Retinitis pigmentosa Cupping in glaucoma (? optic atrophy) Choroidoretinitis Papilloedema **(73)** (also increased size of the blind spot)

CASE 61: HORNER'S SYNDROME

General	**Ptosis** (**75**) / Enophthalmos / Hypohidrosis
Acuity	Normal
Fields	Normal
Pupils	Small (**miosis**) **Reacts** to light and accommodation
Movements	Nystagmus if brainstem disease
Fundi	Normal
Extras	Neck Lymphadenopathy / Scars / Carotid aneurysm Lung Apical "Pancoast" tumour (T1 muscle wasting and sensory loss) Brainstem disease CVA (**19**) / MS (**20**) / Syringomyelia (**84**) Look for sensory loss / Bulbar palsy / Nystagmus (**64**) Idiopathic in young women Ipsilateral carotid bruit (Dissection of artery) Heterochromia of iris (less pigment in affected eye)

Comment

This is an examiners' favourite and you should be aware of the anatomical course of the sympathetic supply to the pupil: Midbrain–Medulla–T1 cord–T1 root–Thoracic ganglion–Ascending preganglionic fibres–Superior cervical ganglion–Carotid plexus–Long ciliary nerve–Short ciliary nerve–Radial pupillodilator muscle / Muscle of Müller.

CASE 62: HOLMES-ADIE PUPIL

General	Young female
Acuity	Normal
Fields	Normal
Pupils	Unilateral **Dilated** (regular) Very **slow reaction** to light and slow returning to resting position Slow reaction to accommodation
Movements	Normal (not if IIIrd nerve lesion – the major differential)
Fundi	Normal
Extras	Decreased or absent ankle jerks Constricts to 2.5% methacholine (no reaction in normals) implies denervation supersensitivity
Points	This is a benign condition. Other causes of a dilated pupil. IIIrd nerve palsy (Ptosis / Looks out) Eyedrops tropicamide / atropine

---

Comment

Small pupils are seen in

- *Old age*
- *Horner's syndrome **(61)***
- *Argyll Robertson Pupil **(63)***
- *Disease in the Pons (CVA etc)*
- *Drugs: Opiates / Pilocarpine eye drops*

CASE 63: ARGYLL ROBERTSON PUPIL

General Bilateral ptosis (frontalis overactivity may make up for this)
Acuity May be decreased if diabetes is cause of ARP
Fields Normal
Pupils **Small irregular**
NO response to light / Normal response to accommodation
"Accommodates but doesn't react" The prostitute's pupil!
Movements Normal
Fundi Optic atrophy if syphilis / Diabetic changes
Points Causes: Neurosyphilis / Diabetes / Pinealomas
Ask to check syphilis serology and urine glucose

Argyll **R**obertson **P**upil = **A**ccommodation **R**eflex **P**reserved

---

Comment

NEUROSYPHILIS *may occur in several different patterns*

Meningovascular *This is a vasculitis that may affect any part of the CNS*

Tabes dorsalis *Dorsal column loss*
Loss of Joint position / Vibration sense / Deep pain
Broad based gait-high stepping / Charcot joints
Bladder insensitivity / Lightning pains / Hypotonia

General paresis of the insane
Dementia / Fits / Tremor – Lips, Tongue

Taboparesis *Tabes dorsalis and GPI with additional upper motor neurone signs (Pyramidal weakness / Extensor plantars)*

CASE 64: NYSTAGMUS

This often causes confusion but in practice there are only a few possible causes. Do not worry about a few jerks at the extremes of eye movement. This is called physiological gaze evoked nystagmus and is normal. Nystagmus nearly always implies **Ear or Posterior fossa disease.**

Nystagmus to one side with greater amplitude in the ipsilateral eye (e.g. Nystagmus on looking right which is most marked in the right eye) is caused by:

> **Ipsilateral Cerebellar** Lesion
> **Ipsilateral Brainstem** Lesion
> **Contralateral Vestibular** Lesion

Cerebellar and **Brainstem** lesions may be Vascular / Neoplastic (primary or secondary) / Demyelinating / Infective.

Vestibular lesions are divided into **Peripheral** or **Central**.

Peripheral	Fast to contralateral side / Fatiguable / Seen on positional testing
	Cochlear dysfunction
	Labyrinthitis
	Menière's disease
	Head injury
	VIIIth nerve disease
	Acoustic neuroma
	Viral neuronitis (Acute vertigo / Nystagmus)
Central	Fast to contralateral side / Not fatiguable / Present at rest
	Vestibular nuclei damage
	Vascular
	Neoplastic
	Demyelination
	Drugs (phenytoin / carbamazepine)

Vertical nystagmus implies central pathology

Upgaze	Level of superior colliculus
Downgaze	Level of foramen magnum

CASE 65: ATAXIC NYSTAGMUS (INTERNUCLEAR OPHTHALMOPLEGIA)

This is a favourite short case. Invariably the patient will have MS and the other eye signs may reflect this.

General	?**MS** (Young / Ataxic speech / Wheel chair) **(20)**
Acuity	
Fields	
Pupils	
Movements	Decreased adduction or lag in adducting eye Nystagmus (fast out) in abducting eye
Fundi	May have Optic Atrophy **(72)**

Teaching Points

Causes	Bilateral	Demyelination (almost always)
	Unilateral	Demyelination Vascular (brainstem ipsilateral to adducting eye)

Comment

The anatomical lesion is in the Medial Longitudinal Bundle ipsilateral to the adducting eye. In many cases bilateral damage has occurred.

CASE 66: IIIrd CRANIAL NERVE LESION

General	Ptosis (complete) / Eye looks out
Acuity	Normal
Fields	Normal but limited by ptosis
Pupil	Dilated (usually no reaction) if complete / Spared if partial
Movements	VIth working – eye moves laterally IVth working – eye intorts on trying to look down and in No other movements if complete but variable movement during recovery
Fundi	Normal / Papilloedema if space occupying lesion

Teaching Points

Causes **Complete (Motor III and Parasympathetic to pupil)**

Sometimes called surgical lesions and often painful

- **Aneurysm** (Ipsilateral Posterior Communicating Artery PCA)
- Tumour

Incomplete (Pupil spared and Ptosis partial)

Nerve trunk infarct	Diabetes (13)
Midbrain lesion	Vascular Demyelination

Comment

There are many other small print causes including encephalitis and parasellar or sphenoidal wing meningiomas. Investigation would include blood glucose, CT or MR brain scan and carotid arteriography.

CASE 67: VIth NERVE LESION

General	No ptosis
Acuity	Normal
Fields	Normal
Pupils	Normal
Movement	Convergent squint at rest No abduction / Reduced abduction beyond the midline Diplopia, worse when looking to the side of the lesion

Teaching Points

Causes
Mononeuritis Diabetes / Sarcoid / SLE **(9)** / Rheumatoid **(8)** / Polyarteritis
Raised intracranial pressure
Brainstem vascular disease
Multiple sclerosis **(20)** (UMN, plaque in pons ? associated VII)
Beware Myasthenia gravis **(99)** if not typical

CASE 68: THYROID EYE DISEASE

General	Exophthalmos / Lid lag / Chemosis
Acuity	Normal (decreased if optic nerve compression)
Fields	Normal (enlarged blind spot if papilloedema)
Pupils	Normal
Movements	Decreased movement not confined to any cranial nerve lesion but superior and medial recti are often the most affected causing variable diplopia (mimicking a IIIrd nerve lesion).
Fundi	Usually normal / Papilloedema if excessive swelling of orbital muscles. Optic atrophy if this is prolonged.

CASE 69: CONGENITAL SQUINT (Strabismus)

The angle between the axis of the two eyes does not change with eye movement.
There is no diplopia.
There may be decreased acuity in the non fixing eye.

When assessing a squint you should perform a cover / uncover test.
Ask the patient to fix his vision on your finger held at arm's length away from his face.
Cover one eye then move your hand to cover his other eye.
The axis of the eye that was first covered will move from its deviated position. The opposite will occur when it is re-covered.

CASE 70: DIABETIC FUNDUS

This is one of the most common short cases in any exam, you should be absolutely sure what you may see and how to present it. Make sure you have seen plenty of diabetic patients during your revision, do not rely on picture books alone.

General	BM stix marks on fingers. Look for these when you are shaking hands.	
Acuity	May be decreased due to macular damage or cataracts.	
Fields	Normal / Central scotoma if macular damage	
Movements	Normal / VIth and partial IIIrd lesions may occur in diabetes	
Fundi	**Background**	Microaneurysms / Blot haemorrhages / Hard exudates
	Pre-proliferative	Microaneurysms / Blot haemorrhages / Hard exudates and Soft exudates + Flame haemorrhages = Ischaemia
	Proliferative	As above plus new vessels esp. disc and macular
	Treated proliferative	Any of the above plus photocoagulation scars Recent = Pale Old = Pigmented

Comment

Treated proliferative is commonly seen in the exam as the signs are usually 'barn door'. After you have finished looking at the fundus try to be bold with your presentation! "This man has treated proliferative diabetic retinopathy as evidenced by the haemorrhages, exudates and laser photocoagulation scars. I would like to examine him for further complications of diabetes and check his blood glucose" ***(13).***

CASE 71: HYPERTENSION

General		
Acuity	Usually normal	
Fields	Enlarged blind spot if papilloedema / Usually normal	
Pupils		
Fundi	Grade I	Arteriolar narrowing / Silver wiring
	Grade II	Arteriovenous nipping
	Grade III	Haemorrhages / Exudates (Soft / Hard)
	Grade IV	Grade III + Papilloedema
	Grades III or IV imply accelerated hypertension	

Comment

Grade III is easy to confuse with preproliferative diabetic changes, but there are usually fewer microaneurysms (dot haemorrhages). Remember that hypertension is a complication of diabetes! If you are in doubt, confess your ignorance and suggest that you check the blood pressure and the blood glucose.

CASE 72: OPTIC ATROPHY

General	? MS (Ataxic speech / In wheelchair)
Acuity	Decreased
Fields	**Central Scotoma (59)** / Bitemporal hemianopia **(57)** if chiasmic compression
Pupils	Normal at rest / **React consensually not directly** (afferent defect Marcus-Gunn pupil)
Fundi	**Pale** Pathological cupping in glaucoma

Teaching Points

Causes

Primary

Damage to nerve

- Optic Neuritis (commonest cause)
- Demyelination **(20)**
- Compression (Tumour / Paget's disease **(101)** / Thyroid eye disease)
- Ischaemic / Toxic (Methyl alcohol / Lead / Quinine)
- Infective (Syphilis) / Nutritional (B12 deficiency **(88)**)
- Hereditary (Friedreich's ataxia **(88)** / Leber's optic atrophy)
- Glaucoma

Secondary

To papilloedema **(73)**

Consecutive

To retinal disease

- Retinitis Pigmentosa
- Choroiditis

CASE 73: PAPILLOEDEMA

General

Acuity Usually normal (may be decreased)

Fields **Increased size of blind spot** / Concentric field loss if severe **(60)**

Pupils Depends on pathology

Movements

Fundi Loss of venous pulsation (early)
Blurred disc margin
Swelling of optic nerve head (localised haemorrhages)
? other signs of hypertensive retinopathy **(71)**

Teaching Points

Causes **Intracranial space occupying lesion**
Tumour / Abscess / Haematoma
Accelerated hypertension
Idiopathic intracranial hypertension
Hydrocephalus
Hypercapnia
Central retinal vein thrombosis
Graves' disease
Hypocalcaemia
Severe anaemia
Guillain-Barré syndrome (Increased CSF protein) Rare

CASE 74: RETINAL PIGMENT

General

Acuity	May be decreased depending on amount of macular damage.
Fields	Variable / Possible central scotoma **(59)**
Pupils	
Fundi	Variable pigmentary changes depending on the cause.

Teaching Points

Race	Dark skin / Pigmented retina
Senile degeneration	Especially macular
Retinitis pigmentosa	Peripheral change first / Widespread if severe Poor acuity / Inherited
Old choroiditis	'Lumps of coal' isolated areas
Laser coagulation	? Other signs of diabetes **(70)**

CASE 75: PTOSIS

Introduce and expose
Observe Drooping of the eyelid
Upper part of iris and pupil covered

Teaching Points

Cause	Other features
IIIrd nerve lesion	Decreased eye movements / Dilated pupil **(66)**
Horner's	Small reactive pupil **(61)**
Idiopathic	Young females **(62)**
Myasthenia	Complex eye movement disorders
Dystrophia myotonica	Balding / Cataract / Myotonia etc **(98)**
Mitochondrial disease	Variable neurological problems (rare)

If ptosis is bilateral, Myasthenia or Dystrophia myotonica are more likely than the other causes.

Comment

The eyelid is kept up by the levator palpebrae superioris which is innervated by the oculomotor (III) nerve (its small superior division) and by the muscle of Müller, supplied by sympathetic fibres (carried along the intracranial blood vessels). There will often be overactivity of the ipsilateral frontalis muscle making the forehead look more wrinkled. If you are not careful you may misdiagnose a contralateral facial nerve palsy.

CASE 76: VIIth NERVE PALSY

Unilateral

Unable to: Close eyes (Eyeball turns up – Bell's phenomenon)
Raise eyebrow (spared in UMN lesion)
Blow out cheeks / Whistle
Show teeth

Facial nerve palsies are divided into complete (lower motor neurone) or incomplete (upper motor neurone).

LMN All muscles of facial expression weak
The nerve is damaged between the nucleus in the brainstem and the face.
By observing whether there is hyperacusis (nerve to stapedius) or loss of taste (chorda tympani) it is possible to say whether the lesion is above or below the facial canal (both preserved if below).

Causes Bell's palsy (Idiopathic)
Cerebellopontine angle tumour **(78)**
Mononeuritis **(86)** esp. Sarcoid / Diabetes
Ramsay Hunt syndrome (Herpes zoster external auditory meatus / soft palate)
Parotid tumour
Middle ear disease
Lesions in the pons Vascular / Demyelinating

UMN The upper motor neurone fibres are damaged between the cortex and nucleus. As there is input from both cortical hemispheres to the upper facial muscles a lesion of one cortex or its tracts will not cause weakness of the upper face. **Upper** Motor Neurone Lesion **Spares Upper** Face.

Causes CVA **(19)**

Bilateral

The differential diagnosis is different as all the causes above are rare bilaterally.

Nuclear	Vascular / Demyelinating
Infranuclear	Guillain-Barré / Sarcoidosis
Muscular	Myasthenia gravis **(99)**
	Myotonic dystrophy **(98)**

CASE 77: CAVERNOUS SINUS SYNDROME

Clinical findings	III IV VI	Subtotal / Total ophthalmoplegia (Painful)
	Vi	Loss of Vi sensation (Ophthalmic division) Loss of corneal reflex
Causes	Thrombosis in the cavernous sinus Tumour (meningioma)	

CASE 78: CEREBELLOPONTINE ANGLE LESION

Clinical findings	V	Loss of corneal reflex Mild weakness of muscles of mastication
	VI	Ipsilateral lateral rectus palsy
	VII	LMN facial weakness Loss of taste anterior 2/3 Hyperacusis
	VIII	Sensorineural deafness
	Cerebellar signs / Nystagmus if large tumour	
Causes	Tumours	Acoustic neuroma / Meningioma (others rarely)

Comment

The CPA is a small triangular fossa between the cerebellum, pons and petrous temporal bone from the Vth to the IXth cranial nerve.

CASE 79: JUGULAR FORAMEN SYNDROME

Clinical findings	IX / X	Decreased palatal movement Absent gag reflex
	XI	Wasting of Sternocleidomastoid Weak head turning to contralateral side Weak shoulder shrugging (upper part of trapezius)
Causes	Tumour Glomus jugulare tumour (Blue eardrum) Fracture at base of skull Paget's disease **(101)** Jugular vein thrombosis	

Comment

Occasionally a large tumour will affect the nearby XIIth nerve in the Anterior Condylar Foramen causing weakness and wasting of the ipsilateral side of the tongue.

CASE 80: BULBAR PALSY

Clinical findings	IX X	Poor palatal movement Loss of gag reflex
	XII	Weak / Wasted tongue / Fasciculation
	Speech	Poor quality / Nasal (as if blocked) due to no soft palate movement
	Cough	Poor cough impulse (may be very feeble) Nasal regurgitation on swallowing (may have nasogastric tube or feeding gastrostomy)

Causes

Motor neurone disease **(83)**
Syringobulbia
Guillain-Barré
Medulla lesions (Vascular / Demyelinating / Tumour)
(Myasthenia gravis **(99)** will produce a similar picture but it is not truly bulbar)

CASE 81: PSEUDOBULBAR PALSY

(UMN lesion) More common than bulbar palsy

Clinical Findings Spastic tongue (Small / Non-fasciculating / Decreased movement)
Poor palatal movement
Gag reflex unreliable, may be lost or brisk
'Donald Duck' speech

Extras **Jaw Jerk brisk** (usually)
UMN signs in limbs
Emotionally labile

Causes **Bilateral CVA (19)** (Internal capsule)
Demyelination
Motor Neurone Disease **(83)**
(Causes upper and lower motor neurone signs in limbs and cranial nerves without sensory signs)
Degenerative cerebral diseases

Comment

It is difficult to tell the difference between these two by just listening. The associated features are better indicators of which type of lesion exists.

...e as asking you to take a history but has the ...irecting you to find out whether there is ...IA, **DYSPHASIA** or **DEMENTIA** (the 3 Ds). Y... establish handedness at some stage. This is better left until near... ...e end but should never be forgotten.

Introduce and expose

Observe Evidence of hemiparesis

Ask *"Please would you tell me your name and where you are"*
If there is obvious dysarthria go on to find whether it is Bulbar **(80)** (Wasted tongue) / Pseudobulbar **(81)** (Brisk Jaw Jerk) or / Cerebellar **(90)** (Nystagmus / Ataxia).
If there is no dysarthria or an inappropriate or incomplete answer test for dysphasia.

Sensory (receptive) *"Please touch your nose"*
"Stick out your tongue"
"Touch your right ear with your left hand"
Speech often fluent but low content

If there is no response or a completely inappropriate response you will be unable to proceed. Tell the examiner *"This patient has a marked sensory dysphasia* (with or without preserved speech). *This would indicate a lesion in Wernicke's area* (with or without Broca's area involvement). *The most likely cause is a CVA. I would like to look for predisposing factors* (hypertension / AF / Bruits etc)".

If there is no sensory aphasia go on to test for motor aphasia

Motor (expressive) *"Would you tell me what this is"* Show the patient your watch / Ask him what the hands and numbers are

If there is a problem this would suggest a lesion of Broca's area. If there is no significant problem go on quickly to test higher cerebral function. You must have a short scheme that is well practised, similar to the following:

Bedside mini mental test

1. Please repeat this address and remember it, I shall test you in a few minutes:

   Mr James Brown
   11 St Andrew's Place
   Regent's Park, London

   If the patient is unable to repeat it back there is a significant short term memory problem.
2. What is the date today (Day / Date / Month / Year) ?
3. Who is the Queen's eldest son?
4. What is in the news at the moment?
5. Add up 3 + 4.
6. Can you tell me the months of the year backwards?
7. What is the difference between a dwarf and a boy?
8. What year did the Second World War start / finish?
9. Finish this – A stitch in time . . . What does it mean?
10. What was the address I gave you?

If everything was normal you missed something!

It is more likely that you will be able to say something along the lines *"This patient has no dysarthria, no/mild motor/sensory dysphasia but he has significant difficulty on a bedside mini mental test indicating loss of higher cerebral function."*

This approach may look long winded at first but if you practise it a few times on your geriatric ward you should find it works fairly smoothly.

NERVOUS SYSTEM
"Examine this Patient's Arms"

Introduce and expose

Observe — Wasting (especially small muscles of hand)
Fasciculation

Arms outstretched
Pyramidal Drift
Winging of scapula

Tone — With the patient relaxed passively flex and extend the elbow, feel for a supinator catch and test for cogwheeling at the wrist.

Power — Test each in turn, always comparing the two sides

	Root Value
Shoulder abduction	C5
Elbow flexion	C6
Elbow extension	C7
Wrist flexion	C7,C8
Wrist extension	C6,C7
Finger extension	C7
Finger spread	T1 (ulnar)
Thumb abduction	T1 (median)

Reflexes — Demonstrate the biceps (C5), supinator (C6) and triceps (C7) jerks. Remember to use *reinforcement* before pronouncing a reflex absent. If reflexes brisk Finger flexion jerks / Hoffman's sign

Sensation — Light touch and pinprick, touch each arm once in dermatomes C4 to T2. Vibration at distal phalanx: if absent wrist / elbow / shoulder.
Joint Position Sense – test using distal phalanx of one finger on each side. If absent, wrist / elbow.

Coordination — Test for Finger-nose incoordination
(Hold your finger at arm's length / No need to move finger)

CASE 83: MOTOR NEURONE DISEASE

Introduce and expose

Observe	**Wasting** especially of the small muscles of the hand / foot **Fasciculation** (Tongue and/or Limbs)
Tone	Normal or increased (spastic)
Power	Either segmental (LMN) or pyramidal (UMN)
Reflexes	Exaggerated (Usually) / Depressed / Absent
Plantar	Extensor / Absent if excessive muscle weakness
Sensation	Normal
Coordination	Normal
Extras	Bulbar **(80)** / Pseudobulbar palsies **(81)**

Teaching Points

Cause	Unknown / 5% familial
Pathology	Degeneration of: Anterior horn cells / Corticospinal tract Motor cortex / Cranial nerve nuclei / Corticobulbar tract
Typically	Age 45–65 / M>F / Mean survival 3 years

Comment

The different proportion of damage to the LMN and UMN in different patients gives rise to a heterogenous clinical picture. Isolated LMN signs are often referred to as Progressive Muscular Atrophy and the corticospinal tract damage as Amyotrophic Lateral Sclerosis (the American term for the whole disease). More often than not both are present giving a mixed picture. Most importantly there should be ***no sensory signs and no bladder symptoms.***

CASE 84: SYRINGOMYELIA

Rare in real life – disproportionately common in exams!

Introduce and expose

Observe	Puffy cyanosed hands Wasting especially small muscles of the hand Scars (from painless burns) Charcot joints Elbow / Shoulder
Tone	
Power	Weakness of segmental (LMN) type – most marked distally Pyramidal weakness below syrinx (lower limbs) **(85)**
Reflexes	Absent in upper limbs / Brisk below (pyramidal tract damage)
Sensation	**Dissociated / Suspended** (normal above and below) **Sensory loss** Loss of Pain and Temperature sensation (Crossing spinothalamic fibres) Preserved Light touch / Joint position sense / Vibration (Uncrossed dorsal column fibres)
Coordination	Normal

Teaching Points

Differential diagnosis	Syrinx Central cord tumour
Associations	Chiari malformation (? downbeat nystagmus **(64)**) Hydrocephalus Horner's syndrome **(61)** Kyphoscoliosis Spastic paraparesis **(85)**

Comment

Syringobulbia refers to syrinx formation in the brainstem giving rise to cranial nerve lesions.

NERVOUS SYSTEM
"Examine this Patient's Legs"

Introduce and expose

Observe Wasting / Fasciculation / Pes cavus / Walking aids / Wheelchair
Foot drop splint

Tone With patient relaxed, gently roll the leg – the ankle should 'flop'
Flex the knee quickly – feel for a 'catch'

Clonus Check for ankle patellar clonus

Power Test each in turn, always comparing the two sides

Activity	Root Value	Main Muscle
Hip flexion	L1, L2	Iliopsoas
Hip extension	S1	Glutei
Knee flexion	L5, S1	Hamstrings
Knee extension	L3, L4	Quadriceps femoris
Ankle dorsiflexion	L4, L5	Tibialis anterior
Ankle plantar flexion	S1	Gastrocnemius

Reflexes Knee jerk (L3/L4)
Ankle jerk (S1)
Remember to use reinforcement before deciding a reflex is absent
Plantar responses (Use an orange stick)

Sensation Light touch / Pinprick
Touch each leg once in dermatomes L2 to S2
Light touch sensation is not always very helpful and sometimes only confuses things, make sure that you are confident in detecting the main patterns of sensory (especially PP) loss (see below).
Vibration at medial malleoli
If absent, knee / iliac crest / sternum
Joint Position Sense (JPS): use big toe on each side
If absent ankle / knee
Hot and cold sensations are carried in the same tracts as PP, testing is therefore omitted.

Diagnoses

- Distal polyneuropathy (Glove / Stocking PP>LT)
- Dermatomal root lesion (PP ≥ LT)
- Spinothalamic loss (PP but not JPS / Vib)
- Dorsal column loss (JPS / Vib not PP)

Coordination Test for heel-shin ataxia

At this stage tell the examiner "At this stage I would usually go on to examine the back for scars, assess the gait and test for Romberg's sign". Hopefully they will stop you and ask you to present your findings.

Gait (91) Ask the patient to walk a short way, turn around and walk back. Be sure to note
Posture / Arm swing / Step size and equality / Circumduction / Ataxia

Romberg's Positive if patient falls when eyes are closed. This implies proprioceptive loss.

CASE 85: SPASTIC PARAPARESIS

Introduce and expose

Observe	Disuse atrophy / contractures - implies long-standing lesion Fasciculation (MND) **(83)**
Tone	Increased - **Spasticity** Ankle and patella clonus
Power	Weakness - flexors / extensors The weakest movements are hip flexion, knee flexion and ankle dorsiflexion
Reflexes	Brisk knee and ankle jerks **Extensor plantars**

The examiner may stop you here - otherwise:

Sensation	Look for a **sensory level** on the trunk, using pinprick sensation.
Coordination	Remember - it will be difficult to assess in presence of spasticity / weakness
Gait	Stiff awkward, 'scissors' gait

Teaching Points

Causes

1. SPINAL CORD COMPRESSION
2. **Multiple Sclerosis**
3. **Motor Neurone Disease**
4. Syringomyelia **(84)**
5. Syphilis **(63)**
6. Sub-acute combined degeneration of cord **(88)**
7. Spinal cord infarction
8. Familial spastic paraparesis
9. Parasaggital lesions
10. Bilateral Cerebrovascular Disease

There are many other, rarer causes.

Comment

Spinal cord compression is the most important to exclude – hence look for sensory level.

In the relatively young patient suspect multiple sclerosis; there may be clues, e.g. cerebellar dysarthria, obvious nystagmus. If you are doing particularly well the examiner may invite you to examine the fundi (optic atrophy), or the upper limbs (finger-nose ataxia). If patient is wearing a collar, and elderly, the likely diagnosis is cervical spondylotic myelopathy (a cause of spinal cord compression).

CASE 86: PERIPHERAL NEUROPATHY

Introduce and expose

Observe	Distal muscle wasting (especially peroneal group) / Footdrop Pes cavus (91) / Claw toes / Charcot joints Callus formation / Skin ulceration (esp. under metatarsal heads) Foot drop splint at side of bed
Tone	May be flaccid if severe weakness
Power	Distal weakness (Ankle dorsiflexion / Plantar flexion / Inversion / Eversion) Eventually also hands
Reflexes	**Absent ankle jerks** (remember to reinforce) Knee jerks absent / Depressed
Sensation	**Loss of pinprick** and light touch in a **stocking** distribution Patchy loss to pinprick more marked distally consistent with a peripheral neuropathy Loss of vibration sense to Knees / Iliac crests / Sternum Loss of JPS at toes
Coordination	
Gait	If weakness of ankle dorsiflexion is prominent, patient may be seen to lift feet up high, before they return to the ground with a 'slap' (**91**).
Romberg's	Should be positive if you have found impaired JPS
Extras	Suggest examining the upper limbs for similar signs and ask to examine the urine to exclude diabetes. Thickened nerves (rare)

Teaching Points

There are very many causes of a peripheral neuropathy, the commonest are
MADD – **M**alignancy / **A**lcohol / **D**iabetes / **D**rugs

A useful summary is: **ABCDEFGH**

Alcohol / **A**myloid
B-vitamin deficiencies
Connective tissue diseases / **C**ancer (but say neoplasia!)
Diabetes / **D**rugs
Everything else!
Friedreich's ataxia
Guillain-Barré syndrome
Hereditary Motor Sensory Neuropathy HMSN (= Charcot Marie Tooth disease)
In 40% no cause is identified, despite full investigation.

Comment

When testing sensation first test pinprick on the thigh, where it will be sharp, then move to the foot. Ask the patient (with his eyes shut) to report when the sensation changes as you move up the leg. Repeat on the medial and lateral aspects of the leg. Repeat for the other leg.

CASE 87: MYOPATHY

Introduce and expose	
Observe	Wasting **proximal** > distal
Tone	Normal
Power	Weakness **proximally** Hip flexion and extension weak / Ankle dorsi- and plantar flexion normal
Reflexes	**Usually normal** (may be depressed) Plantars flexor
Sensation	**Normal**
Coordination	Normal – within the limits of the weakness
Gait	**'Waddling'** Unable to rise from a chair without using hands Unable to rise from crouching position

Teaching Points

Causes
- Inflammatory Myopathies
  - Polymyositis / Dermatomyositis **(47)**
- Metabolic and Endocrine Myopathies
  - Cushing's Syndrome **(92)**
  - Hyper / Hypothyroidism **(93 / 14 / 54)**
- Muscular Dystrophies (dystrophy = genetically determined myopathy)
  - Duchenne / Becker / Myotonic **(98)**
- Polymyalgia Rheumatica
- Paraneoplastic **(3)**

Comment

Remember, all myopathies are proximal, except myotonic dystrophy, and all peripheral neuropathies are distal, except Guillain-Barré syndrome. Other causes of hip flexion weakness may be misdiagnosed if care is not taken. Be sure the weakness is not due to pyramidal disease (85) or to diabetic femoral amyotrophy.

CASE 88: ABSENT ANKLE JERKS AND EXTENSOR PLANTARS

This one is an 'old chestnut'.

If you find absent ankle jerks and sometimes knee jerks together with extensor plantars you will almost certainly be asked for possible causes. The pathophysiology of the findings is:

a) **Damage to the monosynaptic reflex arc** (Peripheral nerve / Dorsal root ganglion / Alpha motor neurone) and therefore reflex loss.
b) **Damage to the corticospinal tracts** leading to an extensor plantar.

Causes

1. Subacute combined degeneration of the cord

Cause	Vitamin B12 deficiency
Pathology	Demyelination of white matter in cord and peripheral nerve
Typically	Patient in 60s / Fair hair / Blue eyes / Pale (Macrocytic anaemia)

2. Friedreich's Ataxia

Cause	Autosomal recessive onset <20 yrs / Autosomal dominant >20 yrs
Pathology	Degeneration of: Dorsal columns / Corticospinal tracts / Cerebellum **(90)** / Spinocerebellar tracts / Peripheral nerves / Dorsal root ganglia
Typically	Young (Male = Female) / Pes cavus **(89)** / Kyphoscoliosis / Dysarthria **(82)**

3. Motor Neurone Disease (83)

4. Syphilitic Taboparesis (63)

5. Combination of two common conditions

Probably the commonest scenario, e.g. an elderly patient with cervical spondylotic myelopathy (producing the extensor plantars) and diabetes (the associated diabetic neuropathy producing the absent ankle jerks).

6. Structural lesion at the conus

The conus refers to the terminal part of the spinal cord (at the level of T12 / L1 vertebral bodies). Within the spinal canal at this point there are many nerves passing downwards before leaving through their appropriate foramina. A lesion within the spinal canal at this level will therefore cause damage to both upper and lower motor neurones.

CASE 89: PES CAVUS

Introduce and expose

Observe **High arched feet**
Clawing of the toes
Associated distal muscular atrophy

<u>**Teaching Points**</u>

Causes Idiopathic
Hereditary Motor and Sensory Neuropathy (Charcot Marie Tooth disease)
Other long standing neuropathies **(86)**
Syringomyelia **(84)**
Old Polio (more likely if Pes Cavus is unilateral)
Spina bifida
Friedreich's ataxia **(88)**

CASE 90: CEREBELLAR SYNDROME

You may be asked to demonstrate some cerebellar signs or on finding one be asked to go on and look for more.

There are groups of signs to look for; from the top down:

Nystagmus	(Lesion is ipsilateral to fast phase **(64)**)
Dysarthria	**Ataxic** (staccato) speech / Ask the patient to say *'British Constitution'*
Finger-Nose ataxia	(Ipsilateral to lesion) with past pointing – Dysmetria
Dysdiadochokinesis	(Poor rapid alternate movements)
Heel-Shin ataxia	
Ataxic gait (91)	Falls to side of lesion

Teaching Points

Causes	Demyelination	MS **(20)**
	Vascular	Posterior circulation stroke **(19)**
	Tumour	In posterior fossa (Primary or Secondary)
	Degenerative	Non-Metastatic manifestation of malignancy **(3)**
		Secondary to Alcohol excess
		Hypothyroidism **(93)**
		Friedreich's ataxia **(88)**
	Primary / Idiopathic	
	Drug toxicity	Phenytoin / carbamazepine

CASE 91: GAIT ABNORMALITIES

If you are asked to examine the gait there are only a few possible outcomes. Once you have recognised the pattern, ask to elicit other signs to confirm your diagnosis.

Spastic The patient walks with hyperextended lower limbs using a scissor like action 'Walking through treacle'. This is due to UMN lesions affecting both legs (**85**).

Hemiparesis One leg is held extended often with a foot drop, the leg is swung out (circumducted) to avoid tripping. Due to UMN lesion on one side (**19**). A similar picture of foot drop can occur with a Common Peroneal nerve palsy but the upper limb is spared.

Cerebellar Broad based gait often falling to one side (**90**).

Sensory Ataxic Foot slapping gait due to loss of proprioception, usually because of Neuropathy (**86**) / Dorsal column loss (Vitamin B12 deficiency / Tabes dorsalis). The patient will have to look at the ground to compensate for the proprioceptive loss.

Parkinsonian Unsteady, small steps, shuffling gait that is difficult to start.
Sometimes the patient is unable to stop. Very unsteady on turning, no arm swing (**97**).

Waddling Seen with muscular dystrophies and other proximal muscle weakness due to loss of control of the pelvis whilst one leg is off the floor (**89**).

THE SPOT DIAGNOSIS

Don't be surprised if, instead of being asked to go through the examination of a system, you are simply asked to look at a patient, or perhaps ask him some questions and then come up with the diagnosis.

Don't panic.

Certain conditions lend themselves to spot diagnosis and tend to come up again and again. Often these are either endocrine or neurological conditions. Most of them should be familiar to you; if not, make sure you recognise them from picture atlases or find them on the wards or in the clinics.

Case Number	
92	**Cushing's Syndrome**
93	**Hypothyroidism**
94	**Acromegaly**
95	**Addison's Disease**
96	**Hereditary Haemorrhagic Telangiectasia**
97	**Parkinson's Disease**
98	**Myotonic Dystrophy (Dystrophia Myotonica)**
99	**Myasthenia Gravis**
100	**Neurofibromatosis**
101	**Paget's Disease**

CASE 92: CUSHING'S SYNDROME

Introduce and expose

Observe Typically Moon face / Plethoric / Acne / Hirsute / Truncal obesity / Wasted limbs / Buffalo hump / Striae / Thin skin with increased bruising / Oral Candida

On recognising a patient with Cushing's syndrome tell the examiner that you would like to perform the following:

1. Measure blood pressure
2. Test for proximal weakness **(87)**
3. Test for glycosuria
4. Ask the patient whether they are taking steroids

Teaching Points

Causes	Iatrogenic	(most often prednisolone)
	Raised ACTH	Pituitary tumour (Microadenoma)
		Ectopic (Small cell lung tumour **(3)**)
	Adrenal tumour	

Comment

Remember Cushing's Disease refers to one specific cause of Cushing's Syndrome, viz. a pituitary ACTH-secreting adenoma. By far the commonest cause of Cushing's Syndrome is iatrogenic, due to the administration of long-term steroids. Hospitals are full of patients on long-term steroids! They may have obvious signs of the underlying disease e.g. Rheumatoid hands, loud wheeze (chronic asthma).

CASE 93: HYPOTHYROIDISM

Introduce and expose in such a way that the patient answers you. You may hear the typical Hoarse / Croaking Voice

Observe	Typically	Female (Middle age / Elderly)
		Overweight
	Face	Coarse facial features
		Peri-orbital puffiness
		Xanthelasma
		Loss of outer third of eyebrows (notoriously unreliable)
		Dry brittle hair
	Neck	? Goitre **(54)**

On recognising hypothyroidism tell the examiner that you would like to ask the patient about specific features of hypothyroidism, look for further signs and any possible predisposing factors.

Symptoms	Cold intolerance
	Lethargy
	Weight gain
	Voice change
	Constipation

Signs	Goitre **(54)**
	Slow relaxing tendon jerks
	Carpal tunnel syndrome **(44)**
	Proximal muscle weakness **(87)**

Predisposing factors

Goitre surgery
Radioactive iodine

CASE 94: ACROMEGALY

Introduce and expose

Observe

Coarse facial features
Prominent supra-orbital ridges
Broad nose
Large jaw / Prognathism (Lower teeth overbite the upper)
Interdental separation increased
Large tongue
Large hands with thick skin
Large head (older examiners may ask about hat size)

On recognising acromegaly tell the examiner that you would like to examine

1. The visual fields / Bitemporal hemianopia **(58)**
   GH-secreting pituitary adenomas are usually large (cf. ACTH- secreting tumours)
2. For evidence of carpal tunnel syndrome **(44)**
3. The urine for glycosuria (Associated diabetes – May have neuropathy etc. **(13)**).

CASE 95: ADDISON'S DISEASE

As this is a little more difficult you may be given a clue e.g. that the patient presented with Malaise / Weight loss / Abdominal pain / Dizziness.

Introduce and expose
Observe Female (young to middle-aged)
Thin
Pigmented skin creases / Mouth / Scars
Postural hypotension
Additional vitiligo **(53)**

It is very common for patients to develop more than one autoimmune condition therefore you may be given the clue that the patient has a history of thyroid disease.

Teaching Points

Other causes of pigmentation are Race, Haemochromatosis, Ectopic, ACTH, Sun tan and Repeated blood transfusions

CASE 96: HEREDITARY HAEMORRHAGIC TELANGIECTASIA

Osler-Weber-Rendu syndrome

This case is very often introduced to the candidate by telling them that the patient presented with anaemia and / or that the patient has a Daughter / Son / Parent with the same problem **(autosomal dominant)**.

Introduce and expose
Observe **Pale** Blood loss (Iron deficiency anaemia)
Lung – Haemoptysis (Bronchiectasis)
Gut – Haematemesis
Telangiectasiae Face / Around the mouth / On tongue and the *undersurface* of the tongue

CASE 97: PARKINSON'S DISEASE

You should be happy to have a case of PD in the exam as the signs are easy to elicit and you will have seen several cases. You may be asked to approach the patient in several ways; examine this man's **Gait (91) / Upper Limbs / Speech / Lower cranial nerves** (facial expression).

Introduce and expose

Observe	Lack of facial expression / Drooling of saliva Poor posture (Stooping / Slumped in a chair) Quiet monotonous speech Slow shuffling gait / No arm swing / Poor balance
Examination	**Bradykinesia (Slow)** moving thumb to other fingers **Rigidity (Stiff)** Best demonstrated at the wrist **Tremor (Shake)** At rest / Often asymmetrical / Pill rolling Power / Reflexes / Sensation usually normal Glabellar tap does not habituate as in normals

---

Comment

L-dopa treatment may lead to chorea / dystonic movements especially of the hands and feet. In contrast to the tremor these movements increase during action.

CASE 98: MYOTONIC DYSTROPHY

You should be able to recognise the facial appearance.

Introduce and expose (May find it hard to release hand shake)

Observe
- **Ptosis** (Uni or Bilateral) **(75)**
- **Myopathic facies** Snarl / Poor smile / Probably unable to whistle
  - Looks Sad / Simple
  - Drooping mouth
- **Temporal Wasting**
- **Frontal Balding**
- **Cataracts** Thick 'coke bottle' glasses

Other features

Myotonia Slow relaxation of muscles
Difficulty releasing grip (worse in cold conditions)
Weakness Especially forearms
Reflexes Decreased
Cardiac conduction defects
Low IQ
Endocrine problems (Small testes / Diabetes **(13)** / Goitre **(54)**)
Autosomal dominant / M>F / Shows anticipation (increased severity with each generation).

CASE 99: MYASTHENIA GRAVIS

Introduce and expose

Observe	Myopathic facies	As **(98)**
	Ptosis	Bilateral asymmetrical / **Fatiguable**
	Eye movements	**Variable strabismus (68)** (diplopia does not fit single nerve lesion) Fatiguable
	Voice	Weak
	Poor swallow	Breathless if very severe (Unlikely in the exam)
	Muscle weakness	Proximal > Distal
	Reflexes	Normal
	No sensory signs	

This is a disease of the neuromuscular junction and may present in the exam for several reasons. Myasthenia may be confined to the eyes with a combination of ptosis, ophthalmoplegia and diplopia, this is similar to thyroid eye disease but there is no exophthalmos and there is ptosis. In addition MG shows fatiguability. If you ask the patient to keep looking up the ptosis will worsen.
Generalised MG is not common but again fatiguability is the hallmark.

CASE 100: NEUROFIBROMATOSIS

Introduce and expose

Observe	Skin Lesions	Cafe-au-lait spots (>5) Axillary freckling Subcutaneous Neurofibromata Mollusca fibrosa (Pink cutaneous fibromas) Plexiform neuroma
	Skeletal	Kyphoscoliosis (50%)

There may be very, very many skin lesions and gross neurofibromatosis can be quite disfiguring.

Eyes	Visual acuity may be decreased due to optic glioma Fundal changes Iris nodules (of Lisch) difficult to see
Hearing	Decreased with acoustic neuroma
BP	Raised if **Renal Artery Stenosis** (Intimal hyperplasia) or more rarely Phaeochromocytoma

Teaching Points

Neurological Complications

Intracranial / Intraspinal / Peripheral nerve tumours
All types of tumour may occur (Glioma / Neuroma Meningioma / Neurofibroma 'A tumour soup')
The signs will be dependent on the location of the tumour.

Comment

There are two types of Neurofibromatosis, both show autosomal dominant inheritance. Positive family history in 50%.

Type I *As described above Von-Recklinghausen's Disease / Chromosome 17.*

Type II *Bilateral VIIIth nerve tumours / No skin or skeletal lesions / Intracranial and Intraspinal tumours also common / Chromosome 22.*

CASE 101: PAGET'S DISEASE

You will be asked to "look at this patient's face" (or legs).

FACE
Introduce and expose

Observe	Increased size of skull Hearing aid

There may be other cranial nerve lesions due to compression as they leave through the many skull foramina

Poor vision / Optic atrophy (Angioid streaks seen on funduscopy)
VIth nerve palsy

LEGS
Introduce and expose

Observe	Bowing of tibia (Anteriorly) Unilateral
Palpate	Warmth (High blood flow)
Auscultate	Bruit

Teaching Points

Complications	Bone Pain / Headache Fractures Poor mobility Nerve / Spinal cord compression Hypercalcaemia Sarcomatous change High output cardiac failure (Rare)

Comment

*The differential diagnosis is of Syphilitic Sabre Tibia and Rickets. Rickets is usually bilateral and syphilis is rare, offer to look for other associated signs **(63)**.*

THE VIVA

The viva can be a very frightening experience as the whole of the medical syllabus is up for discussion. This is usually made worse by your supposed friends who often do their best to 'psych' you out in the days and minutes leading up to the event!

There are a few tips listed below that can make things easier during the exam. There are several ways of gaining valuable experience during your clinical training.

1. Arrange to have a mock viva.
2. Act as a helper if your hospital runs a MRCP course.
3. Ask the consultants who teach you about their favourite viva questions.
4. Ask previous candidates about their experiences BUT get them to remember the common topics as well as the rarities.

During the viva:

- Use good body language (Good eye contact / Hands held on or below table).
- **Speak clearly** / Do not mumble.
- Answer the question asked.
- If you do not understand the question say so at once.
- If you know nothing about the subject under discussion say so at once, either you will be given a clue or the subject will be changed.
- If in doubt about something return to first principles (if you can remember them).
- Make sure you **know about the management of emergency situations** (Cardiac arrest / Acute asthma / Anaphylaxis / Hypovolaemic shock etc.).

When given the situation of an ill person follow this protocol:
Examiner *"You are called to casualty to see a patient who is comatose . . . "*
Candidate *"I would go immediately to the patient and perform*

resuscitation as needed, paying attention to the ***Airway, Breathing*** *and* ***Circulation*** *and I would assess their consciousness level using the* ***Glasgow Coma Scale.***"

This is usually enough for the examiner to set up the case in more detail. *"O.K. He is breathing spontaneously and has a BP of 110/75, HR 85, what would you do next?"*
"I would check his blood glucose and look for small pupils, a sign of opiate overdose."

When asked how you would manage a patient follow this protocol:
"How would you manage a patient with xxxx syndrome?"
"First of all I would confirm the diagnosis by taking a full ***history,*** *performing a complete* ***physical examination*** *and arranging* ***appropriate investigations.***" This shows you would be thorough in your approach to a patient.

Then if you know a specific treatment go on with *"Specific treatment for this condition would be with . . . "*. If you don't know the specifics you could try *"Treatment in general can fall into* ***Conservative / Medical / Surgical / Palliative.*** *In this case Medical drug therapy would be the first option . . ."*.

When asked the causes of a particular condition go through your medical sieve:

VITAMIN-D

V	Vascular
I	Infective (Bacterial / Viral / Fungal / Protozoal / Other)
T	Traumatic
A	Autoimmune / Connective tissue
M	Metabolic / Endocrine
I	Iatrogenic
N	Neoplastic (Benign / Malignant / Primary / Secondary) Neuropsychiatric
D	Degenerative / Ageing

When asked about a particular condition follow a slightly different plan:

Dressed	Definition
In	Incidence / Prevalence
A	Age
Surgeon's	Sex
Gown	Geography
Anaesthetists	Aetiology
Perform	Pathology Macroscopic / Microscopic (Light / Electron)
Deep	Diagnosis Made on **History** **Examination** **Investigation**
Coma	Clinical features Complications (see below)
To	Treatment (Conservative / Medical / Surgical / Palliative)
Perfection	Prognosis

When asked about complications think through each body system in turn:
CVA / RS / GIT / GUT / CNS / Haematological / Immune / Musculoskeletal

As in any exam a degree of luck always helps. We hope your quota arrives for the day! Good luck.

REVISION INDEX